PHILIP L. HILLSMAN, M. D.

Alcohol

DRUGS OF ABUSE
A Comprehensive Series for Clinicians

Alcohol

Norman S. Miller, M.D.
Cornell University Medical College
White Plains, New York

and

Mark S. Gold, M.D.
Fair Oaks Hospital
Summit, New Jersey
and Delray Beach, Florida

Plenum Medical Book Company
New York and London

Library of Congress Cataloging-in-Publication Data

Miller, Norman S.
    Alcohol / Norman S. Miller and Mark S. Gold.
        p.   cm. -- (Drugs of abuse ; v. 2)
    Includes bibliographical references and index.
    ISBN 0-306-43641-8
    1. Alcoholism. 2. Alcohol--Physiological effect. I. Gold, Mark
S. II. Title. III. Series: Drugs of abuse (New York, N.Y.) ; v. 2.
    [DNLM: 1. Alcohol, Ethyl--adverse effects. 2. Alcoholism.
3. Substance Abuse.   W1 DR892 v. 2 / / WM 274 M6485a]
RC565.M4439 1991
616.86'1--dc20
DNLM/DLC
for Library of Congress   91-2391
                                                                  CIP

ISBN 0-306-43641-8

© 1991 Plenum Publishing Corporation
233 Spring Street, New York, N.Y. 10013

Plenum Medical Book Company is an imprint of Plenum Publishing Corporation

Printed in the United States of America

In my judgement such of us who have never fallen victims [to alcoholism] have been spared more by the absence of appetite than from any mental or moral superiority over those who have. Indeed, I believe if we take habitual drunkards as a class, their heads and their hearts will bear as advantageous comparison with those of any other class.

—ABRAHAM LINCOLN

Preface

This book is written for a truly general medical audience. Clinicians, researchers, residents, and students will find *Alcohol* a direct treatment of the major drug problem in America. Along with the first volume in this series on marijuana, *Alcohol* is timely and relevant. The subject is presented with clarity in an effort to provide professionals and interested readers with a basic background in the field of alcohol studies. The emphasis is on what is known and can be counted on as fundamental knowledge on the various aspects of history, epidemiology, diagnosis, treatment, and prevention of alcoholism. Because drugs other than alcohol are such an important feature of the contemporary alcoholic, they are covered as a part of the natural history of alcoholism.

Change and progress are essential to knowledge; past and current research in the alcohol field, as well as detailed discussions of what further needs to be investigated, are included in the volume. The student as well as the practitioner will find the contents useful for didactic purposes as well as a clinical reference. We believe that the researcher will also profit from the comprehensive coverage of the subject. The chapters are organized in sections to highlight important topics and are arranged in a sequence to ensure a logical development of the subject, alcohol. Throughout the book we combine our clinical and research experiences to provide a synthesis that we hope will have widespread clinical usefulness.

N.S.M.
M.S.G.

Contents

1

Introduction and History

The best that history has to give us is the enthusiasm
which it arouses

GOETHE

Alcoholism is less accepted as a disease than mental illness
by the general public and the medical community. Various
forms of mental illness are now considered true diseases;
schizophrenia and manic-depressive illnesses are currently
diagnosed and treated as disorders whose roots are from
biochemical origins in the brain. The evidence for this con-
tention is derived from animal research and response to
pharmacological agents in these disorders.[1]

At the turn of the century and some time after, mental
illness was not viewed as a disease of mind or body. Mental
illness was a moral dilemma for many or a defect or weakness in character, implying a strong volitional component in
the etiology of the mental illness. The source of the em-

phasis on free will was probably based on the observations of the afflicted; they appeared to lack willpower or desire to perform the responsibilities of daily living. The orists such as Bleuer and Kraeplin were keenly aware of the apparent disturbance in will in their descriptions of mental illness and discussions of the pathophysiology of mental illness.[1]

Earlier opinions of mental illness frequently contain references to moral or religious etiologies for it, that is, the devil possessed the sufferer. This notion was not based entirely on imagination as many of the delusions and hallucinations of contemporary forms of mental illness contain references to the devil, persecution, and even god or mythical powers from god. In fact, exorcism in which a specially endowed figure, such as a priest, exorcised the evil spirit that possessed the suffered was an acceptable form of treatment for mental illness in the eighteenth and nineteenth centuries. The important lesson to be learned is that interpretation based on observation is subject to error. Or all that is apparent is not really true.[1]

Alcoholism is in many ways at the stage that mental illness was about 100 years ago. There are signs that alcoholism may also shed the shackles of prejudice, although the progress is not without its significant doubters. Alcoholism is most popularly viewed as a moral problem or defect in character. Correspondingly, the needed treatment is more willpower, generated by self-determination and will. Unaided willpower, however, is doomed to failure in most instances of untreated alcoholism.[2]

The attitude of the physician who has the moral or willpower view of alcoholism is that alcoholism is not an illness that follows known principles of medical science or art. If alcoholism is not a medical disease, then it does not fit the criteria for medical diagnosis and treatment. Furthermore, physicians are reluctant to interfere in the private or religious lives of their patients; because they do not consider alcoholism a disease, physicians do not pursue to identify it in their history and physical examinations. Physicians take a somewhat nihilistic position and do nothing because alcoholism is not a medical disorder and it is lack of willpower.

Modern psychiatry has offered its concepts and methods to solve the mystery of alcoholism. The problems in this approach are manyfold and not entirely the fault of the alcoholic and alcoholism. To begin with, psychiatry is not in total agreement as to how to approach mental illness. There are several schools of psychiatry that offer their own theories, interpretations, and treatments for a particular illness. Each school has its value and application to understanding alcoholism, but the limitations in regard to the diagnosis and treatment of alcoholism are often prohibitive.

Biological psychiatry operates from the assumption that all mental illness originates from a neurochemical basis. This assumption is perfectly reasonable according to our natural laws of the neuroanatomy, neurophysiology and neurochemistry of the brain. One of the major difficulties is that biological psychiatrists use only a few models to understand and treat mental illness. Overextending and overapplying a particular model is not a problem unique to them, of course.

The biologist assumes that depression and delusions and hallucinations are conditions that motivate and sustain the development of alcoholism. The biomedical disorders of affect, particularly, depression, are conditions that "underlie" the alcoholic's need and drive to drink. The alcoholic drinks alcohol to self-medicate or treat the depression. The implication is that the alcoholic is choosing alcohol and alcoholism over a less desirable state of depression. The motivating factor is the depression. Alcoholism is secondary and not etiologic by itself; the etiology is depression. The adherence to "another" condition to explain alcoholism is common among biologists. The biologists do not consider alcoholism to have a neurochemical basis of its own.[5]

Psychodynamic psychiatry has different theories and approaches to alcoholism. The position of these intuitive

scholars is that the psychosocial development and intrapsychic dynamics of the mind are the determinants of the
origin and progression of alcoholism. Alcoholism is an expression of the conflict between unconscious and conscious
forces that produce unbearable and intolerable conditions
for the ego. The ego escapes to alcohol for relief of the disharmonious state. The motivation or drive to use alcohol is
for the tortured ego. Alcohol is secondary and not etiologic.

The "self-medication concept" is not unique to physicians. It is prevalent among lay people and the general public. The usual question is, "Why does he drink the way he
does?" or "Why does she need to drink that way?" The next
sequence is to register reasons for the drinking such as
personal problems, poor childhood upbringing, troubled
marriage, or some other minor or major life problem. The
alcoholic must be drinking because of a series of misunder-
standings and bad breaks. The fundamental idea is that the
alcoholic drinks for reasons outside and not because of internal mechanisms. Alcohol and its effects are not the primary
motivating force for the drinking pattern or behavior. Alcohol always plays a secondary role as an adjunct or bad tool
to manifest the other underlying condition that is "really the
cause" of the drinking.

The self-medication concept is a major obstacle in both
understanding and treating the alcoholic. It always places alcohol as secondary. As long as alcohol occupies a secondary
position, successful recognition and treatment of alcoholism
is severely compromised.

The nature of an addiction to alcohol is such that alcohol
is pursued and is the primary object of concern. The alcohol
is the fundamental trigger and sustaining power behind the
drive to drink. The compulsion to drink alcohol most likely
is derived from a basic interaction between alcohol and the
primitive centers in the brain.

Alcoholism is not a reaction to something else; rather it
is a basic primary drive as powerful as sex or hunger itself

that has been tapped by and associated with the chemical alcohol. The alcoholic continues to drink *in spite of* the developing consequences of the addictive drinking. From this compulsion arises a preoccupation with the acquisition of alcohol that is conscious or unconscious, often the latter. There are frequently times when the alcoholic chooses or wills not to drink but does so anyway in spite of the most fervent decision not to drink. What appears to be a loss of will is really an overpowering of the will to drink that is at the basis of the addiction to alcohol. It is not a lack of will anymore than the drive to have sex or eat is eradicated by willpower or personal resolve. Will or self-control can and does moderate the pursuit and intake of alcohol to some extent, and a measure of control is possible over eating and sexual behavior but not entirely.[4]

Relapse to drinking is inevitable as is "relapse" to eating or a sexual act for most people. There are exceptions, of course. Nature is abundant with exceptions to every natural law and disease. There is, however, a norm or mean set of behaviors that describe most people and most alcoholics. The relapse to drinking for the alcoholic is as natural as any of the other drive states. To not succumb to alcohol is a most unnatural feat that is not ordinarily under the auspices of the unaided will or resolve. The resolve that is used in other matters, that is, answering the alarm clock, arriving to work on time, and the like is woefully inadequate against the basic drives, including the one to drink.

The preoccupation to acquire alcohol, to use it compulsively in spite of adverse consequences, and to relapse or be unable to reduce or eliminate the drinking in spite of the adverse consequences are the essential features of an addiction to alcohol. The pervasive force behind preoccupation, compulsivity, and relapse is loss of control or the inability to overcome the drive to drink. The addiction has a life of its own and is generated by the underlying drive to have alcohol. It does not require other conditions or states to trigger it or sustain it. The psychologists have a theory for drive states that is appropriately applied here. The drive state to drink sets up a tension to drink that is relieved by alcohol as other drive states to eat or have sex are relieved by food or a sexual act. Alcoholics will confirm the tension that is present in a case of untreated alcoholism. The problem with using alcohol to reduce tension from an addiction to alcohol is the loss of control because alcoholism is an aberrant drive to consume alcohol.[4]

The ability to modulate the alcohol may be related to its toxic effects on other parts of the brain. The higher cortical centers that are particularly well developed in man are inhibitory to the lower primitive brain centers where the addictive process lies. Alcohol reduces the efficiency or the inhibitory capacity of these higher cortical centers to control the basic drive to drink. Furthermore, new learning has occurred in the higher cortical centers that needs to be undone or reversed in order for the addictive process to be controlled. This new learning needs to be reinforced regularly.

Still the question lurks in formulation of an understanding of alcoholism: Why do they drink that way? What is wrong? The examination of why people drink is interesting and often productive in understanding normal and abnormal drinking behavior. People drink because they are sad, because they are happy, because someone died or was born, because they were fired or hired, divorced or married, because the job is too stressful or it is going well—in other words, a nearly endless number of reasons are available for why people drink. Not one of them explains addictive drinking. Not one of them accounts for the relentless pursuit and use of alcohol in spite of new adverse consequences. Not one of them is a reason to relapse to alcohol when drinking alcohol could mean disastrous results. The self-medication concept fails as an explanation for alcoholism because it requires that the alcoholic cease using alcohol when it is no longer beneficial. The alcoholic continues to use alcohol long after it is beneficial and is causing adverse consequences.

How does the physician and those who are affected by the alcoholic approach the problem of what to do about the alcoholic and the alcoholism? With all the intuitive knowledge that they have gained with understanding alcoholism? If intuitive knowledge alone were used, then only 3% to 5% of the alcoholics would be diagnosed. That is because only 3% to 5% of alcoholics live on skid row, which is where people think or wish most alcoholics live. This is the physical skid row of the Bowery or wherever cheap alcohol can be obtained and the alcoholic can live a lifestyle of chronic intoxication. The average alcoholic neither lives on nor has visited skid row other than to drive by it, perhaps.[7]

The average alcoholic is married and has a job and a place to live that is miles from skid row. The average alcoholic is in most people's families somewhere or in their place of employment and is around us wherever we go or live. The average alcoholic is not on the verge of catastrophe, although many are by the time they are identified and treated. The average age of onset of alcoholism is in the early twenties for men and women in the United States. Twenty percent of the population is alcoholic, more men than women, although that is changing rapidly.

Other unfortunate positions that the physician takes is that diagnosing and treating alcoholism is none of his or her business. The sanctions and taboos against raising or pursuing the possibility of a drinking problem are staggering. The momentum that must be overcome is enormous. The enabling system that surrounds the alcoholic is large and recalcitrant (an enabler is someone who enables the drinking by allowing, encouraging, or supporting it, or doing nothing about it). All alcoholics have a pervasive and effective enabling system that curiously supports them to continue the alcoholism. The term for the not-too-innocent bystander is *coaddict* or *codependent* because the form and characteristics of the enabling bears strong resemblance to the alcoholic and the alcoholism.[8]

The same denial, minimization, and rationalization are present in the enabler as in the alcoholic so that the enabler is said to be suffering from coaddiction or codependency. The loss of control over the self and the alcoholic is present in the enabler as it is present in the alcoholic. The enabler is as equally unable to make the changes necessary to resolve the coaddiction as is the alcoholic to resolve the alcoholism. Both need education and treatment, whichever applies.

The physician, the employer, the legal system, and much of society at large are enablers for the alcoholism. The major reason is that all of them are using intuitive and archaic methods for diagnosis and treatment. Newer and more effective concepts have not reached them. What is encouraging is that employers and the legal system have made significant changes toward reducing the enabling that is lethal to the alcoholic, those immediately surrounding him or her and the society he or she lives in. The physician, curiously, is lagging behind.

The physician has apparent reasons for enabling the alcoholic. The physician is the advocate of the patient and tries not to give the patient something that is undesirable or untreatable, particularly if it is socially unacceptable. Add this to a recalcitrant enabling system and an angry alcoholic who is in blatant denial of the alcoholism. The final action is to do only what can be done without diagnosing and treating the alcoholism: The physician treats the medical and psychiatric consequences of the alcoholism, which are numerous, in an effort to do something.

Finally, what is common to professionals and nonprofessionals alike is that alcoholism is a personal subject. Everyone has an idea of what alcoholism is that is often intuitive and based on their approach to understanding alcoholism. Many people are affected by alcoholism in a personal way. Because alcoholism is shared by at least 20% of the population in the United States, many people are involved with an alcoholic. Family members, employers or employees, and friends may be alcoholic. Alcoholism is a personal experience for the alcoholic and those affected by the alcoholic. The personal experiences are integrated into how most people view alcoholism. Most people prefer to use these experiences over established criteria for alcoholism. Problems arise in diagnosis and treatment if individual and personal approaches to alcoholism are used. No one would suggest that diabetes or cancer should be diagnosed and treated according to personal pique. Unless alcoholism is taken out of the wrenches of personal prejudice, objective assessment and management are not possible.

Alcoholism is an illness or disease that requires medical diagnosis and treatment. Alcoholism is not a moral problem; rather, moral problems result from alcoholism. Most of what appears to be alcoholism are the consequences of alcoholism. Alcoholism begins simply as an addiction to alcohol that is physical in origin. From the pursuit, compulsivity, and relapse to alcohol, mental, medical, psychiatric, and spiritual consequences ensue. The essential core of the alcoholism needs to be identified so that the consequences will abate. Treating only the consequences will serve to distract the attention from the primary disease of alcoholism and enable the consequences to continue.[3,6,1,9]

Mental illness has reached the correct status of inclusion in the domain of medicine, but alcoholism is not yet a medical disease as medicine is practiced. Although the American Medical Association has officially accepted alcoholism as a disease, its members still struggle with that decision. Approximately 25% to 50% of a general medical practice is composed of alcoholics, according to surveys. The problem is not likely to go away.

Medicine has room for more advancement. In this book, we will attempt to examine why the problem of alcoholism is so large and why the medical profession with many others continues to struggle in relative blindness for a solution that already exists.

References

1. Kaplan HI, Sadock BJ: *Synopsis of Psychiatry: Behavioral Sciences Clinical Psychiatry*, 5th Ed., Baltimore, Williams and Wilkins, 1988.
2. Jellinek EM: *The Disease Concept of Alcoholism.* New Haven, CT, College and University Press, in association with Hillhouse Press, New Brunswick, NJ, 1960.
3. Vaillant GE: *The Natural History of Alcoholism: Causes, Patterns and Paths to Recovery.* Cambridge, MA, Harvard University Press, 1983.
4. Helzer JE, Robins LN, Taylor JR *et. al*: The extent of long-term moderate drinking among alcoholics discharged from medical and psychiatric treatment facilities. *N Eng J Med*, 1985; 312:1678-1682.
5. Guze SB, Cloninger R, Martin R, Clayton PJ: Alcoholism as a medical disorder, in *Alcoholism and Outcome*, Rose, RM, Barrett, J, eds.: New York, Raven Press, 1988.
6. Gordes B: Guest editorial: The disease concept of alcoholism. *The Psychiatric Hospital*, 1989; 201:151–152.
7. Adams RP, Victor M: *Principles of Neurology*, 3rd ed. New York, McGraw-Hill, 1985.
8. Miller NS, Millman RB: A common cause of alcoholism. *J. of Substance Abuse Treatment*, 1989; 41–43.
9. Milam JR, Ketcham, K: *Under the Influence.* Seattle, WA, Madrona Publishers, 1981.

2

Prevalence and Pattern of Use

Count not the cups; not therein lies excess in wine,
but in the nature of the drinker.

MENANDEY, Fragment

Alcoholism is much more common than most people, including physicians, think. Most people are reluctant to consider that alcoholism is a common disorder because of the peculiar stigma that is attached to it and the tenacious denial attendant to those who have alcoholism and those who do not. Also, the tendency to assign alcoholism to another disorder makes the alcoholism disappear in definitions only to reappear in an atypical or perplexing diagnosis. The medical profession and the public are reluctant to accept that drinking alcohol carries with it significant risk to develop a degree of loss of control over its use. Loss of control leads to myriad adverse consequences that are stereotypical and predictable for alcoholism which make it possible for alcoholism to be diagnosed.

The criteria for determining the prevalence of alcoholism vary greatly from study to study, from decade to decade, from country to country, and from discipline to discipline. The criteria for alcoholism today are by no means universally agreed upon. Professional and personal preference, experience, orientation, and bias continue to plague attempts to construct useful and applicable criteria for the diagnosis of alcoholism. Difficulty in reaching unanimity is not unique to the field of alcoholism but is more pronounced and the consequences more serious.[1,2]

Epidemiology of Alcoholism

In spite of these problems in ascertaining prevalence and patterns of use, there do exist several surveys on alcohol use and one diagnostic survey that do make significant attempts to ascertain the prevalence of alcoholism and reflect the extent of its use in the United States and other parts of the world. The important surveys are performed or supported by the National Institutes on Drug Abuse (NIDA) or National Institute on Alcoholism and Alcohol Abuse (NIAAA). The NIDA surveys are the (1) "Drug capsule," which is a survey on use of alcohol and drugs by high school seniors; (2) the National Household Survey, which examines the use of alcohol and drugs by the U.S. population at large; and (3) the Drug Abuse Warning Network (DAWN), which monitors the emergency rooms in hospitals throughout the United States. The NIAAA surveys concern (1) the use of alcohol by vulnerable populations defined as alcoholics or others who stand to lose by consuming alcohol and (2) the use in the general population that pertains to the health and medical complications of alcohol use and alcoholism.[3,4]

Another major epidemiological study obtained data on the actual prevalence of the diagnosis of alcoholism from five major cities in the United States and three major cities elsewhere in the world. A major contribution of this study was to use criteria for the diagnosis of alcoholism that were not bound by medical consequences. This study is a milestone in the quest to derive useful epidemiological findings on the prevalence of alcoholism. The study also provided useful information on the prevalence of the existence of other psychiatric disorders that either are a result of the effects of alcohol and alcoholism or coexist with alcoholism to aggravate it or vice versa, that is, the alcoholism undermines diagnosis and treatment of the psychiatric diagnosis.

Some of the most interesting statistics pertain to who uses alcohol and how they use it. Most Americans drink alcohol. Reliable surveys indicate that 90% of Americans have had a drink of alcohol at some point in their lives. According to the most rigorous study, about 16% of the population suffers from alcoholism. However, 80% or more of the alcohol consumed in the United States is consumed by the alcoholic. In other words, only 16% of the alcohol consumed in the United States is done so by 80% of the population. Alcoholics are a devoted and dedicated lot when it comes to consuming alcohol.

The target population can be further characterized by recognizing that the onset of alcoholism in the United States for males is 22 years and 25 years for females. Interestingly, this age gap is narrowing as more women are becoming alcoholic and doing so at a younger age. These findings suggest that alcoholism is a disorder of the young and not the old as is the popular myth. The image of the elderly skid-row drinker is a distorted fantasy that exists in a fraction of reality. Skid-row alcoholics comprise only 3% of the alcoholics in the United States, and many of them are younger than is commonly recognized.[5]

Where do we find the alcoholic? According to most

studies and clinical experience, the typical alcoholic is white, black, or other, has a job, is married, and has achieved any level of education. It is important to remember here that half of the alcoholics are older than 22 years old for men and 25 years old for women. The racial breakdown indicates that alcohol knows no racial barriers—the lifetime rates of alcoholism are about the same for whites, blacks, and others.[5,6,7]

The rate of alcoholism among occupations does tend to be more common among the less skilled, but this may represent a phenomenon of "downward drift" in which the alcoholism retards the acquisition of education and skills. The prevalence of alcoholism according to levels of education does not confirm higher rates of alcoholism among the less educated. Because the onset of the first symptom of alcoholism is commonly between the ages of 15 and 19 years, it is not surprising that job development is impaired in the critical formative years when decisions are made and performances that have far-reaching consequences are judged. Even so, the rate of alcoholism is 16.3% for alcoholics completing somewhere between 0 and 7 elementary grades, 11.1% for those completing Grade 8, 18.3% for those completing 9–11/GED, 12.8% for high-school graduates, 13.8% for college level, and 10% for college graduates. The majority of alcoholics have at least a high-school education or equivalency.[5]

Alcoholics are most likely to marry or cohabitate. Although 8.9% percent have a stable marriage, 29.2% cohabitate. Only 15% never married, and 40.4% have had at least one divorce or separation. The major consequence of alcoholism is a disruption in the interpersonal relationships; therefore it is easy to see why so many alcoholics have problems in their marriages.[5]

The prevalence of alcoholism is equal for white and blacks at 14% lifetime prevalence, and 17% for Hispanics. A further analysis reveals that white and black women are also equal at 5%. Hispanic men have a higher rate of alcoholism at 30% and Hispanic women lower at 4%.

The lifetime prevalence of alcoholism according to geography is also interesting. The rates of alcoholism are higher among the urban dweller than among rural or suburban dwellers as a lifetime prevalence rate of 15% is found in Baltimore, St. Louis, and Los Angeles and 11% in Durham and New Haven.

Another interesting set of figures is that when heavy or problem drinkers are considered as a group, the number of men who fulfill criteria for alcoholism is only 50%. This means that an additional 23% of men drink often and heavily but are not alcoholic by the criteria in this study. Thus a total of 50% of the male population drinks problematically. The proportion of women who are alcoholic among heavy drinkers is 35%. Clearly, drinking is a common event, and problem drinkers are also common.[5]

The age groups that predominate in prevalence of alcoholism are 18–29 years in white men and women, whereas 45–64 years is the age for black men and 30–44 for Hispanic men. For women, both white and Hispanic women peak at 18–29 years, and black women like black men peak at 45–64 years.[5]

The duration of alcoholism is also relatively predictable. Alcoholism tends to be a progressive illness overall with a steady deterioration in personality and health over time. According to the studies, the mean duration of alcoholism is 9 years for those who eventually experience a remission of 1 year or more. Because the mean age of alcoholism is in the early and middle twenties, the typical duration of alcoholism is between 1 and 5 years, followed by 6 to 10 years in duration. This is in contradistinction to the popular conception that the typical alcoholic is old and a long-time drinker. What is very interesting is that alcoholism can and does develop within a year as 17% of those in remission from alcoholism for more than a year were alcoholic within 1 year from the onset of the drinking histories.[5]

These findings are enlightening for the understanding of the diagnosis and treatment for alcoholism. The importance of early diagnosis and treatment is clearly suggested by the data. The majority of the alcoholics are diagnosable and treatable by 5 years after the onset of drinking. This is so because the distribution of the duration of alcoholism is skewed toward the shorter duration of alcoholism. A small but significant number report a duration of greater than 10 years with a large range between 10 and greater than 50 years. The mode or most frequent duration is 1 to 5 years and almost 50% of those who report a remission of alcoholism for greater than a year experienced a duration of alcoholism 5 years or less.[8,9]

The diagnosis of alcoholism can be made earlier in the natural history of the disease than most have suspected. Effective treatment for alcoholism does exist so that earlier intervention is desirable. Many of the medical complications that are usually relied on for the diagnosis occur later in onset; although they are reliable indicators of adverse consequences of alcoholism, medical complications are not particularly sensitive earlier in the course of alcoholism. The behavioral criteria describe the loss of control over alcohol that leads to the adverse consequences in disruption in interpersonal relationships. The manifestations of the disruption in interpersonal relationships is in marital, legal, employment, and other areas of the alcoholic's life.

Any discussion of the younger alcoholic of today is remiss without attention being given to the prevalence of other drug use along with alcohol. The alcoholic under the age of 30 years old, which constitutes the majority of the alcoholics today, is addicted to at least one other drug in addition to alcohol. The most common drug is marijuana, followed by cocaine, sedative/hypnotics, hallucinogens, and others. Reversing the index drug: Of those who are addicted to marijuana, 36% are alcoholics; of those who are addicted to barbiturates, 71% are alcoholics; of those who are addicted to cocaine, 84% are alcoholics; of those who are addicted to opioids, 67% are alcoholics.[5]

The contemporary alcoholic is a multiple drug addict who combines and substitutes one drug for another. In a history session during a medical evaluation, this observation must be utilized in order for an accurate diagnosis to be made and correct treatment to be instituted. Carefully planned detoxification schedules are based on accurate histories and diagnoses. Also, prescribing practices must be modified to take into account the vulnerability alcoholics have for other drugs, particularly, sedative/hypnotics and tranquilizers. Alcoholics became easily addicted to a wide variety of drugs, presumably because of generalized vulnerability to drug and alcohol addiction.[10,11]

The locations where alcoholics can be found are well known but useful to summarize. The household contains an alcoholism rate of 14%. This means that 1 out of 6 people living in households will suffer from alcoholism at one point in their lives, most likely early in their lives. Among men, 1 out of 4 will suffer from alcoholism and among women, 1 out of 12 will suffer from alcoholism.[12,13]

The prevalence of alcoholic patients seen in clinical practice is common, especially, in view of the fact that alcoholics are overrepresented among patients seen in clinical practice. Approximately 25% to 50% of patients in a general medical practice is composed of alcoholics. A general medical practice is defined as consisting of the typical household, in any class population, with no predominance of a particular illness. The consequences of the alcoholism are commonly hypertension, gastrointestinal problems, upper respiratory illness, cardiac complaints, trauma, and other abnormalities.

Because a general medical practice is devoted to a large number of chronic-care patients, it is not surprising that the proportion of alcoholics in such a practice is so high. The prevalence of alcoholism is 14.4% among chronic-care patients, defined as chronic illnesses. Some of the chronic illnesses are a consequence of alcoholism, others are not. Certainly, alcoholism aggravates or contributes to the severity, course and prognosis of the chronic illness.[5]

A not too surprising figure is that the prevalence of alcoholism among the psychiatric population is as high as 50%. Alcoholism itself produces psychiatric symptoms so that many of these patients have alcoholism as the primary problem. The diagnosis and treatment of alcoholism in many instances will resolve the psychiatric symptoms. However, the correct diagnosis of alcoholism must be made before proper treatment can be instituted.[14]

The prevalence of alcoholism among the incarcerated is alarmingly high. Fifty-seven percent of those incarcerated qualify for the diagnosis of alcoholism. Approximately half of them have had active alcoholism in the past year. Other well-known statistics are that over 80% of murders involve someone who was intoxicated with alcohol at the time of the murder. Eighty percent of domestic violence involves someone who was intoxicated at the time of the violence. More than 50% of automobile deaths involve someone who was drinking.

If these statistics seem alarming to some, it might be because the previous epidemiological studies did not ascertain diagnoses. The most recent, comprehensive epidemiological study from which the data in this chapter was derived is the first to use diagnostic criteria, the *Diagnostic and Statistical Manual III* (DSM-III). The ECA (Epidemiological Catchment Area) data actually diagnosed alcoholism and did not estimate it. The criteria from the DSM-III were derived from other operationally defined criteria that have been used extensively in research protocols. The DSM-III criteria have a universal application and have been verified in clinical trials. The criteria describe addictive use, tolerance, and dependence. The most critical addition is the criterion for addictive use. These criteria reflect the loss of control over alcohol that is central to the diagnosis of alcoholism as recommended by the World Health Organization. Tolerance and dependence are not specific for alcoholism as they occur in normal drinkers who do not demonstrate alcoholism or the loss of control over alcohol. Also, younger, healthier alcoholics do not show significant tolerance and dependence as do older, more chronic alcoholics.

Prior to the DSM-III criteria, the rates of alcoholism were not based on diagnoses; rather estimates of alcoholism were based on (1) excessive consumption; (2) the social and health problems that are a consequence of excessive consumption, and (3) alcohol dependence, characterized by the development of physical tolerance and/or dependence.

A formula that estimates the number of alcoholics in the population from cirrhosis death rate is inexact because there is no fixed ratio of alcoholism to liver cirrhosis as the formula must assume. Cirrhosis death rates per capita consumption are aggregate statistics that can only be used to estimate overall rates in large populations. Aggregate statistics do not measure the severity, frequency of occurrence, personal characteristics associated with alcoholism, or its risk factors such as age, sex, or the presence of other disorders.

Alcoholic beverage sales are used to calculate the average per capita consumption of the population; however, per capita consumption does not predict the prevalence of alcoholism. There is not a known correlation between per capita consumption and the prevalence of alcoholism, that is, a low rate of alcoholism may be associated with a high proportion of abstainers. Or, as is the case in the United States where a high rate of alcoholism is associated with a high proportion of moderate drinkers, the per capita consumption is supported by a minority of heavy drinkers and alcoholics in the population, although they are substantial in number.

Even these studies with their inherent deficiencies have demonstrated a prevalence of alcoholism to be between 7% and 12%. The ECA data are based on personal interviews of 20,000 people in five major cities in the United States. The same DSM-III criteria were used for all the subjects. The demographic variables were collected in the same fashion in a standardized way in all the locations. Objective and sophisticated statistical analysis was used to analyze the data as well.

The conclusions that can be derived from the epidemiologic data confirm what clinicians have suspected and researchers have documented for some time. Alcoholism is the most common psychiatric disorder in the United States. Over their lifetimes, nearly 16% of adults have diagnosable alcoholism, and half of these have been in the active stage in the past year. Men are about five times as likely as women to suffer from alcoholism, but the gap between the two is closing. For both men and women, the onset of alcoholism is in the early and middle twenties.

Although alcoholism is prevalent in all ethnic groups, the increase in the black/white ratio of lifetime prevalence with increasing age is particularly interesting. Education does not seem to be a distinguishing factor, and although all occupations are represented, less skilled positions are overrepresented by alcoholics as possibly a downward drift due to the consequence of alcoholism.

Pharmacological dependence is not a good criterion by which to diagnose alcoholism because a lower proportion are dependent. Presumably this is at least partially so because the duration of alcoholism is, on the average, 9 years and almost 50% of the alcoholics have the onset of alcoholism before 5 years of alcohol consumption.

Self-recognition of excessive drinking appears to be prominent. The majority of alcoholics recognize they are consuming more than they should but are very often unwilling to share this self-awareness in a therapeutic setting. Careful evaluations by those who come into contact with alcoholics more than any other, namely the physician, are needed.[5]

References

1. Robins LN, Helzer JE, Croughan J, Ratcliffe KS: The NIMH Diagnostic Interview Schedule: Its history, characteristics, and validity. *Arch. Gen. Psychiatry* 1981; 38:381–389.
2. Robins LN, Helzer JE, Weissman M, Ovaschel H, Gruenberg E, Burke J, Regier DA: Lifetime prevalence of specific psychiatric disorders in three sites. *Arch. Gen. Psychiatry* 1984; 41:949–958.
3. Johnston ID, O'Malley DM, Bachman JA: *Use of Illicit Drugs by America's High School Students: National Trends 1975–1984.* DHHS Pub. No. (ADM) 85, 1394, Washington, DC, U.S. Government Printing Office, 1985.
4. Miller JD, et al.: *National Survey on Drug Abuse: Main Findings.* Rockville, MD, NIDA. 1985.
5. Robins LN, Helzer JE, Przybeck TR, Regiev DA: *Alcoholism in the Community: A Report from the Epidemiologic Catchment Area. Alcoholism: Origins and Outcomes.* Rose R, and Barrett J, eds. N.Y., Raven Press, 1988.
6. Bell RA, Schwab JJ, Lehman RL, Traven ND, Warheit GJ: An analysis of drinking patterns, social class and racial differences in depressive symptomatology. In Seixas, FA, ed.: *Currents in Alcoholism.* New York, Grune & Stratton, 1978.
7. Robins, LN: *Alcohol abuse in Blacks and Whites as Indicated in the Epidemiological Catchment Area Program,* pp. 63–75, in Danielle Spiegler, ed., *Alcohol Use Among U.S. Ethnic Minorities.* Proceedings of a Conference on the Epidemiology of Alcohol Use and Abuse Among Ethnic Minority Groups, September 1985. DHHS Publication No. (ADM) 89–1435. Printed 1989.
8. Polich JM, Armor DS, Braiker HB: *The Course of Alcoholism.* Santa Monica, CA. Rand.
9. Regier DA, Myers JK, Kramer M, Robins LN, Blazer DG, Hough RL, Eaton WW, Locke BZ: The NIMH Epidemiologic Catchment Area (ECA) Program: Historical context, major objectives and study population characteristics. *Arch. Gen. Psychiatry* 1984; 41:931–941.
10. Myers JK, Weissman MM, Tischler GL, Holzer CE, Leaf PJ, Orvaschel H, Anthony JC, Boyd HJ, Burke JD, Kramer M, Stoltzman, R: Six-month prevalence of psychiatric disorders in three communities. *Arch. Gen. Psychiatry,* 1984; 41:959–967.

11. Miller NS, Mirin SM: Multiple drug use in alcoholics: Practical and theoretical implications. *Psychiatric Annals* 19: 5 May, 1989.
12. Greenblatt M, Schuckit MA: *Alcoholism Problems in Women and Children.* New York, Grune & Stratton.
13. Winokur G, Clayton PJ: Family history studies, IV. Comparison of male and female alcoholics. *Q J Stud. Alcohol* 1968; 29:885–891.
14. Shapiro S, Skinner EA, Kessler LG, Van Korff M, German PS, Tischler GL, Leaf PJ, Benham L, Cottler L, Regier DA: Utilization of health and mental health services: Three epidemiologic catchment area sites. *Arch. Gen. Psychiatry* 1984; 41:971–989.
15. Miller NS, Gold MS: Suggestions for changes in DSM-IIIR Criteria for substance use disorders. *American Journal of Drug and Alcohol Abuse* 1989; 15(2):223–230.

3

Genetics of Alcoholism

Drunkards beget drunkards...

PLUTARCH

Alcoholism in Families

One observation is relatively certain: Alcoholism runs in families. Medical experts seem to agree on this point more than any other. Any given alcoholic has a 50% chance of having at least one family member with alcoholism. A family that has at least one alcoholic is likely to have others, that is, 90% chance of having two or more family members with alcoholism. Furthermore, alcoholics with a family history of alcoholism tend to have a more severe course with greater adverse consequences from alcoholism. Alcoholic parents have alcoholic children about 4 to 5 times more often than do parents who are not alcoholics.[1,2,3]

The Bible contains references to families with drunkards. Aristotle and Plutarch pondered it, and doctors and preachers of the Nineteenth century were adamant that drunkards beget drunkards. Alcoholism was a weakness or vice to most of them that was inherited like any other talent or lack of it.

No other psychiatric illness has as strong a familial dominance. Schizophrenia and affective illness have a family representation greater than expected in the general population but not as frequent as alcoholism. Some neurological conditions exceed alcoholism in incidence rates within families such as Huntington's Chorea, in which a particular offspring has a 50% chance of developing the disease if a parent is affected. The probability of a child's developing alcoholism is 25% if a parent is alcoholic. The probability is greater than 50% if both parents are alcoholics.[4,5]

Why the confusion about alcoholism if heredity plays such a large role for so many? Estimates place the rate of alcoholism in the United States between 10% and 20%. That means somewhere between 20 and 40 million Americans suffer from alcoholism. We all know at least one person, often a family member, who is alcoholic.

Researchers in recent times have used a variety of techniques to arrive at the same conclusion that alcoholism is inherited rather than determined by environment. By the 1970s the debate between the nature/nurture approaches diverged. Although many agree that alcoholism ran in families, it had not been decided if environment or upbringing was more, less, or as important as genetics. This natural antagonism is present in many other psychiatric disorders, for example, schizophrenia. If environment is the culprit, then modification of practices and behavior is indicated. If heredity is the determining cause of alcoholism, then the problem originates in a physical predisposition that initiates alcoholism.[8,9]

The research approaches used by medical investigators have been interesting and challenging to understand. Basically, the designs of the studies have been to try to isolate heredity from environment. The studies have come relatively close, but no one type of study has been able to yield the entire answer to the question of nature versus nurture. Even so, the evidence is convincing that heredity plays by far the largest role in alcoholism. The studies have examined twins, adoptees, families, and offspring of alcoholics.[6]

Twin Studies[7–13]

Researchers in Sweden, Finland, and the United States have found greater concordance of alcoholism among identical twins than among fraternal twins. The assumption is that the inheritance is stronger in identical twins because they have genes or genetic endowments that are identical. Fraternal twins, on the other hand, share only about half of their genes.[1–3]

Environment still cannot be eliminated because twins reared in the same environment are treated similarly, so in effect they are subject to the same environment. Even genetically different offspring might have an effect that makes them both alcoholic if environment is responsible for the development of alcoholism.[5]

Adoption Studies

The research on adoptees is interesting because it eliminated environment substantially, more than any study to date, but not completely. In Denmark, a study found that the biological parent and not the foster parent determined whether the adopted offspring developed alcoholism. The adoptees were adopted at the age of 6 months from the biological mother. The 9 months in the uterus and the first 6 months of life were still under the influence of the biological mother so that environment was not entirely controlled for. However, the remaining years, into adulthood, were under the environment of the adopted, foster parents.[3] In this milestone study, the adoptees who became alcoholics had biological parents who were alcoholic much more often than foster parents who were alcoholic. Furthermore, even if the foster parents were alcoholic, the adoptees without an alcoholic biological parent did not become alcoholic.[1,2,4-17]

The biological parents share genes with the adopted-out offspring so that the hereditary background of the adoptee was the determining factor in the transmission of alcoholism. The environment of the alcoholic did not play much of a role in the development of alcoholism in the adoptees. Even in homes where alcoholism was active, if the offspring did not share the genes for alcoholism with the rearing parent, then no alcoholism in the offspring was present. In the study, probability of becoming an alcoholic was about 25% if the biological father is alcoholic. This is true whether the child is a son or daughter. The number of mothers who were alcoholic was too small in this study to make such predictions.

When heredity and environment factors are both present and operating together, the transmission of alcoholism is still very strong. As might be expected, the probability of having a family history positive for alcoholism is greater if both heredity and environment are influences on the children. The probability of having a first-degree relative (father, mother, sister, or brother) who is alcoholic is at least 50%.

Researchers became weary as they tried to unravel the cause of alcoholism by studying alcoholics. The problems are many because of the pharmacological effects of alcohol on people, especially, if the alcohol is consumed often and in large amounts. Researchers wanted to know if the greater tolerance for alcohol that alcoholics show was acquired or inherited. Tolerance is defined, in this case, as being able to have more alcohol without much effect of the alcohol. Someone who has increased tolerance for alcohol seems to be able to drink large quantities without showing the effects, that is, getting as drunk as quickly. Alcoholics appear to have this enhanced tolerance early in their drinking histories, perhaps, *before* the onset of their alcoholism.[18]

High-Risk Studies

Studies have also examined the children of alcoholics. The children who had not yet started to drink much and who had not yet developed alcoholism were ideal candidates to use. These children are called "high-risk" individuals because their positive family history of alcoholism places them at higher risk to develop alcoholism than individuals without a family history of alcoholism.[19,20]

Tolerance to alcohol was studied in these children before they became alcoholic. Tolerance was measured objectively and subjectively. Motor coordination and thinking abilities were scored in children with and without a family history of alcoholism. The children who had an alcoholic parent were able to perform better on tests of motor coordination and thinking than children who did not have a parent with alcoholism. Furthermore, as would be expected among those possessing greater tolerance, the high-risk children reported that they did not feel as intoxicated with the same amount of alcohol as did the matched low-risk children.[21-23]

What these results tend to show us is that alcoholics may indeed inherit an ability to drink more than others without the genetic predisposition to develop alcoholism. The reason that alcoholics early in their drinking histories drive everyone else home may be that they react differently to alcohol. The brain in alcoholics is probably "wired" in a way that tolerance is greater for alcohol than someone without the genes for alcoholism. The location for tolerance is in the brain and not the liver where the metabolism or breakdown and elimination of alcohol occurs. The liver does increase the rate of breakdown of alcohol but not substantially enough to account for the total amount of tolerance.

Tolerance

Tolerance is a "physical" sign and symptom that is inherited and not some personality factor such as low self-esteem or inferiority complex or other deep-rooted psychological problems. The predisposition to alcoholism begins as a physical reaction to alcohol that is called *tolerance*. Those with a low risk for alcoholism do not adapt well to the presence of alcohol in their brains. The reactions of the lack of tolerance is dysphoria or a disturbed mood, nausea, headache, maybe vomiting, and general ill feeling that only gets worse with more alcohol. The nonalcoholic actually feels better as the alcohol leaves the body so there appears to be little reinforcement to drink more alcohol. The alcoholic, on the other hand, feels better as the blood-alcohol level rises in the body and brain so that the motivation is to drink more.

This negative reaction or low tolerance to alcohol can also be inherited. Orientals and some Occidentals have an intolerance to alcohol that is manifested as a "flushing reaction." The Oriental flushing reaction appears to be inherited. The reaction is characterized by dysphoria, headache, nausea, vomiting, lightheadedness, and a red flushing over the face and sometimes body. An Oriental with the flushing reaction usually has several members of the family who also have the same reaction to alcohol.[24]

The rate of alcoholism among Orientals is low, and this intolerance to alcohol may be a protective mechanism against alcoholism. This is an example of a genetic predisposition against alcoholism that is also physical. The families of Orientals who have this "flushing reaction" have a lower rate of alcoholism than families without the protective "flushing reaction."

Tolerance to alcohol or the lack of it appears to be inherited. Whether someone is likely or not to develop alcoholism appears to depend on whether or not he or she has the genes for alcoholism. If someone has tolerance for alcohol, he or she may be at risk for developing alcoholism. The opposite may be true; if someone lacks tolerance to alcohol, he or she probably will not develop alcoholism.

There are other markers of alcoholism in addition to tolerance. The electroencephalograph (EEG) and other instruments that also measure brain-wave activity have been used to find some interesting differences between children of alcoholics and other children without alcoholic parents. High-risk subjects show more slow alpha activity after consuming alcohol than low-risk children. Also, children of alcoholics show slower onset and progression of other waves, for example, P waves when measured in the absence of alcohol. These waves may be important in thinking and how fast someone reacts in thinking.[25,27]

The exact interpretation of these findings is unclear at this time. The important conclusion now is that the brains of alcoholics may be different from the start, even before birth, as determined by the genetic makeup.[25-27]

The Role of Environment

Caution is urged as there are always exceptions and factors other than genes that are important in the development of alcoholism. Environment, with its many and complex interactions with the genetic makeup, is important in the expression of alcoholism. Tolerance to alcohol may be a necessary condition but not always a sufficient condition for alcoholism to occur. A particular kind of environment may be more conducive to alcoholism for some personalities than others.

A simple and convenient way to view heredity and environment is in an equation in which the predisposition to alcoholism plus the exposure to alcohol equals an addiction to alcohol or alcoholism. Heredity, as discussed, creates the physical predisposition to alcoholism. The exposure is defined by the broad concept of environment. There are many determinants of exposure to alcohol, beginning with the practices, customs, norms, and laws within a given culture. Most cultures, including those in the United States, have a high tolerance for alcohol. Alcohol is relatively cheap, easy to obtain, a fixed tradition in religious and social practices, and its use is even encouraged and enforced by groups within our society. The powerful media of television, magazines, and roadway billboards inundate and saturate all ages, at all times, in all places. Almost no one can escape the exposure to alcohol with varying degrees of overt and tacit approval and disapproval regarding its use.

When the physical predisposition is present, even in varying degrees of vulnerability (which may be the case with alcoholism as it is with many other genetic disorders such as diabetes mellitus), exposure is required to develop the disease of alcoholism. The intensity of the exposure may vary as may the duration, so that someone will drink much and often in certain environments (for example, in college or certain employments, such as bartending) or not so much or often in others. As a rule of thumb, the more the genetic loading (i.e., both parents being alcoholic) and the greater and longer the exposure, the more likely that alcoholism will develop. Contrariwise, the absence of a family history with little exposure is least likely to develop alcoholism. Any combination of either heredity or environment will determine the risk for the development of alcoholism.

We all know exceptions to this rule, for example, someone with a host of alcoholics in the family who is not alcoholic, or someone who is alcoholic but does not have a single relative with alcoholism. The reasons for these exceptions may be (1) little opportunity for exposure to alcohol, (2) denial of alcoholism in the family, that is, mother or grandfather had a "nervous breakdown," (3) misattribution of alcoholism to another illness, for example, depression (alcoholism causes depression), (4) nonpenetrance of the alcoholism in a particular generation as does occur in genetic disorders, and (5) the theory, or some of it, can always be incorrect.

The "Addictive Personality"

No one kind of "addictive" personality appears to predict alcoholism. An addictive personality appears to develop in the setting of alcoholism and probably as a consequence of alcoholism. The addictive personality does not seem to be inherited or to be present before the onset of alcoholism.[28]

However, some types of personalities seem to be at high risk to develop alcoholism. Antisocial behavior in childhood frequently leads to alcohol drinking and eventual alcoholism. A high proportion of those with antisocial personalities suffer from alcoholism. It is estimated that somewhere between 50% and 90% of those incarcerated in prisons are alcoholic, and many of those are antisocial personalities.[29]

Summary

Every study shows that the strongest predictor of future alcoholism is a family history of alcoholism. About one of every 4 or 5 children of alcoholics in North America and Western Europe becomes alcoholic in all the studies. Alcoholism runs in families. The reason is genetic constitution. Environment is important but plays a different role than the cause, more like contributing to the probability to the development of alcoholism if the genes for alcoholism are present.[30,31]

References

1. Goodwin DW: Alcoholism and genetics. *Archives of General Psychiatry* 1985; 42:171–174.
2. Goodwin DW, Schulsinger F, Hermansen L, Guze S, Winokur G: Alcohol problems in adoptees raised apart from alcoholic biological parents. *Archives of General Psychiatry* 1973; 28:238–243.
3. Goodwin DW, Schulsinger F, Moller N, Hermansen L, Winokur G, Guze SB: Drinking problems in adopted and non-adopted sons of alcoholics. *Arch General Psychiatry* 1974; 31:164–169.
4. Goodwin DW, Guze SB: *Psychiatric Diagnosis.* New York, Oxford University Press, 1984.
5. Schuckit MA, Haglund, RMJ: An overview of the etiologic theories on alcoholism. In Estes N, Heinemann E (Eds.): *Alcoholism: Development, Consequences, and Interventions.* St. Louis, MO; Mosby, pp. 16–31, 1982.
6. Miller NS, Gold MS: Research approaches to inheritance of alcoholism. *Substance Abuse J* 1988; (3):157–168.
7. Schuckit MA: Biological vulnerability to alcoholism. *Journal of Consulting and Clinical Psychology* 1987; 55(No. 3):301–309.
8. Cloninger CR, von Knorring AL, Sigvardsson S, Bohman M: *Inheritance of Alcohol Abuse.* Paper presented at the International Conference on Pharmacological Treatments for Alcoholism: "Looking to the Future," organized by the Alcoholism Education Centre and the Institute of Psychiatry, University of London, England, March, 1983.
9. Cloninger CR, Reich T, Yokoyama S: Genetic diversity, genome organization, and investigation of the etiology of psychiatric diseases. *Psychiatric Developments* 1983; 3:225–246.
10. Kaij L: *Studies on the Etiology and Sequels of Abuse and Alcohol.* Lund, Sweden, University of Lund, 1960.
11. Partanen J, Bruun K, Markkanen T: Inheritance of drinking behavior: A study on intelligence, personality, and the use of alcohol of adult twins. In Pattison EM, Sobell MB, Sobell LC (eds.): *Emerging Concepts of Alcohol Dependence.* New York, Springer Publishing Co., Inc., 1977, Chap. 10.
12. Murray RM, Clifford C, Gurlin HM: Twin and alcoholism studies. In Galanter M, ed.: *Recent Developments in Alcoholism.* New York, Gardner Press, 1983, vol 1, chap. 5.
13. Hrubec Z, Omenn GS: Evidence of genetic predisposition to al-

coholic cirrhosis and psychosis: Twin concordances for alcoholism and its biological end points by zygosity among male veterans. *Alcoholism Clin Exp Res* 1981; 5:207–215.

14. Schuckit MA, Goodwin DW, Winokur G: A half-sibling study of alcoholism. *Am J Psychiatry* 1972; 128:1132–1136.

15. Bohman M: Some genetic aspects of alcoholism and criminality: A population of adoptees. *Arch Gen Psychiatry* 1978; 35:269–276.

16. Bohman M, Sigvardsson S, Cloninger R: Maternal inheritance of alcohol abuse: Cross fostering analysis of adopted women. *Arch Gen Psychiatry* 1981; 38:965–969.

17. Cadoret RJ, Cain CA, Grove WM: Development of alcoholism in adoptees raised apart from alcoholic biologic relatives. *Arch Gen Psychiatry* 1979; 37:561–563.

18. Goodwin DW: Alcoholism and genetics. *Arch Gen Psychiatry* 1985 (Feb.): 42.

19. Schuckit MA, Engstsrom D, Alpert R, Duby J: Differences in muscle-tension response to ethanol in young men with and without family histories of alcoholism. *Journal Of Studies on Alcohol* 1981; 42:918–924.

20. Schuckit MA: Studies of populations at high risk for alcoholism. *Psychiatric Developments* 1985b; 3:31–63.

21. Schuckit MA: Ethanol-induced changes in body sway in men at high alcoholism risk. *Arch Gen Psychiatry* 1985a; 42:375–379.

22. Schuckit MA: Subjective responses to alcohol in sons of alcoholics and controls. *Arch Gen Psychiatry* 1984c; 41:879–884.

23. Schuckit MA: Differences in plasma cortisol after ethanol in relatives of alcoholics and controls. *Journal of Clinical Psychiatry* 1984b; 45:374–379.

24. Chan AW: Racial difference in alcohol sensitivity. *Alcohol and Alcoholism*, 1986; 21:193–204.

25. Begleiter H, Porjesz B, Bihari B, Kissin B: Event-related brain potentials in boys at risk for alcoholism. *Science* 1984; 227:1493–1496.

26. Gabrielli WF, Mednick SA: Intellectual performance in children of alcoholics. *Journal of Nervous and Mental Disease* 1983; 171:444–447.

27. Gabrielli WF, Mednick SA, Volavka J, Pollock VE, Schulsinger F, Itil TM: Electroencephalograms in children of alcoholic fathers. *Psychophysiology* 1982; 19:404–407.

28. Vaillant GE: *The Natural History of Alcoholism*. Cambridge, MA, Harvard University Press, 1983.

29. Cloninger CR, Bohman M, Sigvardsson S, von Knorring AL: Psychopathology in adopted-out children of alcoholics. In Galanter M, ed.: *Recent Developments in Alcoholism* (pp. 37–51). New York, Plenum Press, 1984.
30. Goodwin DW: Studies of Familial Alcoholism: A Review. *Journal of Clinical Psychology* 1984; 45(12):December.
31. Cadoret RJ, O'Gorman TW, Troughton E, Heywood E: Alcoholism and antisocial personality: Interrelationships, genetic and environmental factors. *Arch Gen Psychiatry* 1984; 42:161–167.

4

Neurological Effects of Alcohol

Drink drives out the man and brings out the beast.

ALBERT CAMUS

The analysis of the anatomy and physiology of the brain explains a lot about the myriad of effects of alcohol on behavior. The various locations of the brain serve as areas of specific functions for behaviors. These behaviors, in turn, are directly attributable to certain anatomical designations in the brain. A systematic understanding of the physiology of the brain further explains the action of alcohol and other drugs on the brain to produce certain patterns of behavior.[1,2]

Cerebral Effects

The higher centers of the brain are located in the cerebral cortex. This is a phylogenetically new portion of the brain that is especially developed in humans in comparison to lower animals. The frontal, temporal, parietal, and occipital lobes do not have sharp demarcations for their borders, but rather show a gradual transition from one lobe to the other.[1,2]

The frontal lobe contains the nerve cells for the important functions of judgment, propriety, social and individual values, ability to plan, initiative and drive, abstraction, and language function. The frontal lobe provides inhibition of instinctual drives such as sex, appetite, thirst, and hunger and controls the sense of right and wrong, the herd instinct for social integration, the organizational capacity to formulate and execute complex plans, fine motor functions of the arms and legs and face and trunk, and the abstraction of arithmetic and verbal symbols of language. A variety of neurological and psychiatric syndromes result from disruption of the function of the frontal lobe from any cause.[1,2]

Surgical lobotomies are directed at portions of the frontal lobe, specifically, the cingulate gyrus, to reduce the initiative and drive from aggression and obsessive-compulsive disorders. Dementia or senility from any cause, particularly, Alzheimer's disease, includes a loss of the abilities of abstraction, planning, propriety, social and personal interactions, and initiative. The destruction of the left posterior frontal gyrus produces an interruption in language function (expressive aphasia), a disturbance in the production of everyday language exhibiting decreased output, misnaming, and poor repetition of words on command. Aphasia is commonly seen in stroke, less in dementia and brain tumors.[1,2]

During acute intoxication from alcohol, similar impairments in frontal-lobe functions are seen. Judgment is impaired, motor coordination is awkward, abstraction and concentration are limited, acts of impropriety and short-sightedness are common, and language is incoherent and disconnected.

Eventually, after regular and addictive alcohol use, initiative and drive are lessened, antisocial acts are increasingly present, compromising of values are disturbingly frequent, and a sustained and progressive plan for living is increasingly difficult. Abstraction and concentration are more disturbed as the time of continued consumption of alcohol widens. Tremors and other incoordination of motor movements begin to appear as chronicity of drinking expands.[3]

The parietal lobe contains more subtle functions but not any less important to overall neurological and psychological functioning. The functions of the parietal lobe are visual spatial orientation, abilities to recognize objects by touch, intuition, melody perception in music, and denial. Disturbances in parietal lobe function produce fascinating syndromes in neurology and psychiatry that include abnormalities in judging the orientation and position of body parts in space, the recognition of body parts belonging to the individual, intuition, and melody. Patients who have experienced a stroke that involves the parietal lobe will not be able to dress one half of their body, usually the left, because of a denial that it exists. Also, a complete paralysis of an arm and leg may be denied. The sense of knowing where in space a body part may be is lacking so that awkward accidents may occur in walking and using arms. The intuition that is so necessary to formulating good conclusions is disrupted, reducing the individual's capacity to react to everyday living with a rhythm and flow that is smooth and efficient.

Alcohol in acute and chronic use produces many of the abnormalities that are attributable to parietal lobe dysfunction. A sense of detachment of the body and the self, known as depersonalization, often occurs. The self is aware of the body from a distance in an objective and strangely detached feeling. The fluid intuitive state is frozen, making logical and coherent thinking difficult. Uncoordinated and awkward expression of body movement is common. These impairments from alcohol are subtle, hard to measure, and mixed with emotions and perceptions.

The temporal lobe contains diverse functions for memory, hearing, and language. Recent or short-term memory is located in the hippocampal gyrus of the temporal lobe. The acquisition of new memory traces is dependent on retention in short-term memory before consolidation, and registration in banks for long-term memory can occur. Short-term memory for words and language is located in the left temporal lobe for most individuals; nonverbal information, that is, symbols and sensations, is retained in the right temporal lobe.[1,2]

Alcohol has a predilection for the hippocampus, often producing defects in recent memory. Alcohol does not actually erase memory; rather, it prevents the formation of memory traces by interfering with the acquisition of new memory in the hippocampus of the temporal lobe. A blackout is the lack of formation of new memory. During a blackout, there is no recollection of the events occurring during intoxication because no memory was recorded in the presence of alcohol. Faulty memory during periods of intoxication is due to frequent blackouts. Blackouts are significant because they represent loss of control over the use of alcohol.

The temporal lobe is the location of the termination of the nerves for hearing. The cortical representation of hearing is located in Heschel's gyrus of the temporal lobe. It is not clear how alcohol can specifically affect hearing, but it is known that people do not hear as well while intoxicated and frequently raise their voices because of the lack of modulation of the feedback of the volume of the speech.[2,4]

The reception of language is located in the left temporal lobe for most individuals. Chronic users of alcohol appear to have difficulty understanding or listening to what is being said to them.[2,4]

The occipital lobe processes visual information. Visual acuity is impaired during acute and chronic intoxication. One's ability to discern objects and motion is reduced (blurred vision). The effect of chronic use of alcohol is to blunt hues of colors and sharpness and designs and patterns that are perceived. Alcohol's effect on the occipital lobe is the specific reason for these aberrations in vision.

Intelligence is a collection of the functions of the various lobes of the brain. The association areas are broad connections between the lobes and lower brain functions that will be discussed later in this chapter. Long tracts of fibers of nerve cells run from the frontal lobe to the temporal lobe, which then sends connecting fibers to the occipital lobes. There are a few major association areas, such as the frontotemporaloccipital, frontotemporoparietal, temporoparitoccipital, and so forth. The association areas summate and integrate brain functions to coordinate the complex brain functions that comprise intelligence. The function of intelligence is to learn, and it requires the mental capacities of abstraction, memory, association, and logic. The capacity for judgment in the frontal lobe is not acting in isolation. It is connected to recent memory stores in the temporal lobe and can access visual images in the occipital association area. Working together results in the intelligence to inhibit a thought or a drive and to refrain from acting on an impulse to drink that might enter the conscious.

Alcohol interferes with proper function of the association areas, thereby adversely affecting intelligence. Measurement of intelligence confirms that as little as 2 ounces of 80-proof whiskey or vodka will reduce the intelligence quotient by a substantial amount. The IQ scores of alcoholics at the time of active consumption of alcohol are significantly less than months after a protracted period of abstinence from alcohol. Researchers have determined that the IQ scores of alcoholics continue to improve for as long as 1 year after stopping drinking. The areas of intelligence that are commonly affected by chronic alcohol consumption are abstractions, memory, judgment, and planning.[3]

The "brain damage" that recovered alcoholics frequently refer to in a humorous way is probably true in most instances. However, this reduction in IQ is often reversible over a prolonged period of time, covering months and years. Alcoholics commonly experience an improvement in their intelligence years later as they achieve a greater ability to remember, to abstract, and to judge. The reason for the impairment in IQ is not clear as a single cause. Alcohol is a toxin that is known to kill nerve cells so that a direct effect of alcohol may account for the brain damage. Additionally, some drinkers may have a vitamin deficiency, particularly, vitamin B complex that contains thiamine or B1, niacin, pyridoxidine or B6, or B12. These vitamins are important in the preservation and functioning of nervous tissue.[5,6]

Any deficiency can result in nerve damage that is manifested in an observable behavioral change. Thiamine deficiency produces Wiernicke–Korsakoff's syndrome. The initial presentation of Wiernicke's syndrome is a confusional state, with ataxic or uncoordinated gait, nystagmus or jerky eye movement, and ophthalmoplegia or a paralysis of eye movements and peripheral neuropathy. All aspects of the syndrome improve with thiamine administration.

After the confusion clears, Korsakoff's syndrome will emerge in some patients. Korsakoff's syndrome is a loss in the ability to make new memory with the other intellectual faculties reasonably well preserved. Individuals with this syndrome can calculate, recall past events, and carry on logical and coherent conversations but cannot remember the name of the person or gist of the conversation taking place. Korsakoff's syndrome improves with thiamine, but normal memory does not always return. Korsakoff's can be seen in conditions other than chronic alcohol use in which malnourishment has occurred and a less-than-minimum requirement of thiamine has been taken.[6,7]

Pellagra is another syndrome that is characterized by a dementia, diarrhea, dermatitis, and death. The missing vitamin is niacin. This condition is not seen in the United States as much as in other Third World countries where niacin deficiency is more prevalent.[6,7] Toxic amblyopia or blindness due to optic nerve damage occurs in some chronic alcohol drinkers because of a lack of vitamin B12.[6,7]

Many drinkers and alcoholics today do not develop these rather severe syndromes, although substantial numbers continue to appear on the wards of the inner-city hospitals and the state hospitals. Improved nutrients, earlier diagnosis, overall better health status, and more carefully regulated distilling practices account for fewer cases of these specific syndromes.

Limbic Effects

The next major level of the brain is the limbic system, composed of a number of diverse brain structures in a cooperative arrangement for the execution of a variety of related functions. The structures that comprise the limbic system are the cingulate gyrus of the frontal lobe, the hypothalamus, septal area, thalamus, amygdala, and hippocampus. These structures form the Papez circuit. The limbic system is one of the oldest portions of the brain phylogenetically and has remained relatively constant over the centuries of evolution from lower animal forms to the present-day man.[2]

The functions of the limbic system are primitive, as is suggested by its persistence in anatomy and physiology in the animal kingdom from early evolutionary history. This fact has profound implications for the theory of addiction as it may be as old as evolution, at least, in animal forms comparable to man. The addiction to alcohol as well as other drugs, food, and perhaps other substances and behaviors may originate in the drive states that are located in the limbic system. These drive states are for food, thirst, and sex; they are otherwise known instincts.

Mood and memory are also located in the limbic system. Anxiety, depression, anger, affection, and other shades of emotions have been traced to the various limbic structures. Stimulation of the septal area in man and animals produces rage, sexual orgiastic pleasure with erections, and mounting behavior in animals. Destruction of the cingulate gyrus in man and the amygdala in animals produces placid and acquiescent behavior.[2]

Brain Stem Effects

The brain stem is the next area below the limbic system. The structures of the brain stem are (from top to the bottom), the midbrain, pons, and medulla. The midbrain is home of the reticular activating system (RAS) that is responsible for maintaining wakefulness and alertness. A sleeping mother is able to hear a baby's cry because of the stimulation of the RAS. Any disturbance to the RAS will result in an alteration in consciousness, usually, a loss of alertness, sleepiness, and even coma.[2]

The pons is important for behavior as it is the location of the locus ceruleus, which is composed of nerve cells that contain the neurotransmitter, norepinephrine. Norepinephrine is an important neurotransmitter in the function of the autonomic nervous system that is responsible for the fight-or-flight reactions as well as other vital functions such as heart and blood pressure.[1,2]

The medulla consists of centers for the regulation of the heart rate, blood pressure, and respirations. These medullary centers for vital functions are ordinarily autonomous and spontaneous in firing. Disturbance to these centers may result in life-threatening consequences with a decrease and even cessation of vital functions.[1,2]

The acute effects of alcohol are predictable and identifiable in a descending pattern of depression of brain function. The brain is affected more noticeably than other organs. In the brain, alcohol is largely a depressant but in low doses has an apparent stimulant effect. The exhilarating effect of alcohol is known to many but is largely a subjective effect. On objective measurements, alcohol has essentially exclusively depressant effects.[3]

Central Nervous System

The most sensitive portions of the brain are the highly integrated centers such as the cerebral cortex and the reticular activating system. The cerebral centers that are responsible for memory, concentration, and insight are affected early by low amounts of alcohol (such as an ounce or less), worsening progressively with higher blood levels of alcohol. Personality changes with an enhanced and expansive mood and emotional displays and swings that may fluctuate from laughter and giddiness to sadness and tearfulness. The ability to modulate the emotions is impaired. Effusive outflow of emotions may quickly and suddenly alternate between affectionate affect, sometimes thick, to angry, intimidating displays.[3]

The mood is equally as vulnerable to the effect of alcohol as dysphoric reactions are common in low doses in some individuals and in many at higher doses. Depression may be associated with depressive thoughts, even self-destructive to the idea of suicide. Negative attitudes and decisions are frequently encountered as the effect of alcohol persists with continued intake. The effect on mood is a result of the perturbation by alcohol of the limbic system and the cerebral cortices. A frank lowering of the mood with a sad effect, feelings of lack of appreciation of pleasure and of interests in self-concern is reflective of a disturbance in the limbic system. A cognitive set of impending doom, self-worthlessness, lowered self-esteem, and hopelessness is a reflection of a disturbance in the cerebral hemispheres.[8-11]

In general, the effects of alcohol on the central nervous system (brain) are proportional to blood-alcohol concentrations. As the alcohol blood level increases, the areas of the brain are affected in a progression of descending "paralysis," beginning with the outer cerebral hemispheres, moving through the limbic system, brain stem from the midbrain, through the pons and finally the medulla.

The reason for the differential sensitivity of the various brain locations is the different neuronal networks that comprise these areas. The highly resistant brain stem areas contain the polysynaptic pathways that are needed to protect the vital functions. The cerebral hemispheres lack these dense, highly integrated, interwoven network of neurons and their fibers.[3]

Although alcohol has this anesthetic property and can produce unconsciousness, the margin of safety is minimal for use in surgery. A requirement for being a good anesthetic agent is to provide a sufficient dose range of safety in the surgical plane III of anesthesia where surgery can take place with analgesia and muscle relaxation and usually loss of consciousness. Alcohol has a narrow range of blood-alcohol levels for the surgical level of anesthesia, so that the next surgical plane IV of high morbidity and mortality is quickly reached, where the loss of blood pressure, pulse, and respirations occur.[3]

When the descending paralysis reaches the midbrain in high enough blood concentrations, the level of alertness and consciousness is comprised with sedation and sleep. The RAS is normally resistant to low and moderate blood levels of alcohol; however, at high alcohol levels, the center of wakefulness is dulled and eventually suppressed to absent functioning that results in coma. Coma is a state of irreversible sleep unless the causing agent is removed.[3]

The pons, the center for eye movements, is affected so that when alcohol reaches sufficient concentrations, the eyes do not move in the unconscious state (the patient must be unconscious to involve the pons in a descending paralysis). Also, the pupils become pinpointed in size in the locked and fixed position at the pontine level.[3]

The medulla is the last stop for the descending paralysis by alcohol. The vital functions are severely affected and in high enough concentrations of alcohol are arrested. Blood pressure is not maintained, the heart ceases to beat, and respiration stops. Life cannot be sustained without mechanical intervention, and death will result from an arrest of vital functions. Within a few minutes, death to the brain begins to spread through the sensitive areas until the necrosis is completed.[3]

The reason why lethal overdoses are not common is because a large enough bolus must reach the medulla to suppress vital functions before unconsciousness occurs. In descending paralysis, alcohol reaches the midbrain before the medulla to suppress the reticular activating system that is responsible for consciousness. In the unusual circumstance, someone, usually young and daring, is able to consume a large dose of alcohol in time for it to reach the stomach before unconsciousness occurs. The alcohol continues to be absorbed into the bloodstream after the RAS in midbrain has been saturated with enough alcohol to produce sleep. That is why it is imperative to lavage the contents of the stomach in a suspected overdose of alcohol, when the intoxicated person cannot be aroused after vigorous physical stimulation.[3]

The electroencephalograph provides an objective measurement of the changes that are occurring in the brain. The earliest recognizable change from the acute effect of alcohol is the slowing of the normal alpha rhythm and the appearance of low waves in the theta range, followed by delta waves that are slower waves.

References

1. Adams RP, Victor M: *Principles of Neurology,* 3rd ed. New York, McGraw-Hill, 1985.
2. Isaacson RL: *The Limbic System.* 2nd ed. New York, Plenum Press, 1982.

3. Ritchie JM: The aliphatic alcohols. Chapter 19, pp. 372–386. In *The Pharmacological Basis of Therapeutics,* eds. Gilman AG, Goodman LS, Rall TW, Murad F. New York, Macmillan Publishing Co., 1985.

4. Danbe JR, Sondok BA: *Medical Neurosciences: An Approach to Anatomy, Pathology and Physiology by Levels.* Boston, Little, Brown, Co., 1978.

5. Petersdorf RG, Adams RD, Braunwald E, et al. (eds.): *Harrison's Principles of Internal Medicine,* 10th ed. New York, McGraw-Hill Publishers, 1983.

6. Lieber CS: *Medical Disorders of Alcoholism,* Philadelphia, W.B. Saunders Co., 1982.

7. Mendelson JH, Mello NK: *The Diagnosis and Treatment of Alcoholism,* 2nd ed. New York, McGraw-Hill, 1985.

8. Parsons OA, Leber WR: The relationship between cognitive dysfunction and brain damage in alcoholics: Causal, interactive, or epiphenomenal. *Alcoholism* 1981; 5:326–343.

9. Schuckit MA: Alcoholism and affective disorder: Diagnostic confusion. In Goodwin DW, Erickson CK, (eds.): *Alcoholism and Affective Disorders.* New York, SP Medical and Scientific Books, 1979, pp. 9–19.

10. Mayfield DG: Alcohol and affect: Experimental studies. In Goodwin DW, Erickson CK, eds.: *Alcoholism and Affective Disorders.* New York, SP Medical and Scientific Books, 1979, pp. 99–107.

11. Katchadourian HA, Lunde DT: *Fundamentals of Human Sexuality,* 3rd ed. New York, Holt, Rinehart & Winston, 1975.

5

Medical Complications
of Alcoholism

All sorts of bodily diseases are produced by half-used
minds.

GEORGE BERNARD SHAW

The medical complications of alcoholism are important for
physicians to know in detail. However, as important as medical sequelae can be, the majority of alcoholics escapes irreversible medical consequences. The minority of alcoholics
who have medical consequences appears to represent a
chronic, longtime consumer or one who has an idiosyncratic
reaction to the effects of alcohol.[1,2,3]
    The medical consequences are related to a host of organ
systems in the body. Ethanol is water soluble and reaches
virtually every cell that is bathed by water. The toxic effects
of ethanol on the body are both direct and indirect. Studies

47

have confirmed that ethanol produces direct toxic damage to organs, for example, brain and muscle, and also influences the development of deficiency states through malnutrition or metabolic derangement.[4]

The major organ systems affected are the cardiovascular, gastrointestinal, hematologic, oncologic, respiratory, integumentary, traumatic, endocrinologic, and neurologic. These organ systems are regularly affected by measurable means although less often to significant pathological extents. The individual susceptibility appears to vary considerably, and explanations are not always available to predict who will develop which complications.[1-4]

Cardiovascular System

A common complication from acute and chronic alcohol consumption is an elevation of blood pressure and pulse. After acute administration of alcohol, the physiological response to the elimination of ethanol is a discharge of the sympathetic nervous system with a concomitant rise in blood pressure and pulse. The development of sustained hypertension and tachycardia are common sequelae of regular and chronic alcohol consumption.

An elevation can be detected during the intoxicated state and especially in the early abstintent state while the blood-alcohol level is either dropping or was recently zero. The absolute values for blood pressure and pulse may or may not be in the abnormal range, depending on the individual reaction to alcohol withdrawal. Those who are young and without existing hypertension are less likely to have an elevation than those who are older and predisposed to some hypertension.[5-7]

An elevation in the first 24 to 72 hours of 20 to 30 mm Hg in systolic blood pressure and 10 to 20 mm Hg in diastolic blood pressure over baseline for a particular individual is typical following chronic consumption. The values are lower for withdrawal from acute ingestion. The pulse is elevated 10 to 30 beats per minute, in the range of sinus tachycardia after heavy and more chronic consumption of alcohol.

The blood pressure often returns to normal over a period of a few days without specific therapy. It is important to realize that individuals with an elevation in blood pressure and a history of chronic alcohol consumption have acclimated to the sustained increase. These individuals should be allowed to have blood pressure and pulse gradually subside in the abstinent state with or without specific medical intervention.

A vast majority of those alcoholics with an elevation in blood pressure and pulse will turn out to be normotensive. The remainder who continue to have some degree of hypertension will require less medications while in the alcohol-abstinent state. Elevated blood pressures, often in the hypertension range, occur with a high prevalence. Any patient with hypertension and tachycardia should be assessed for alcohol intake and alcoholism.

Alcoholic cardiomyopathy is probably more common than currently considered because of underdiagnosis of alcoholism in general, particularly in medical populations. A significant proportion of the "idiopathic cardiomyopathy" heretofore attributed to a viral ideology almost certainly have an alcohol-induced basis.[8,9]

What is generally known about patients with cardiomyopathy (underdiagnosis notwithstanding) is that a chronic drinking history of at least 10 years, especially with heavy intake, is noted. The signs and symptoms of cardiac insufficiency from cardiomyopathy are generally gradual in onset, although precipitous occurrences have been reported. Patients present most often with heart failure, manifested by breathlessness, fatigability, palpitations, anorexia, and dependent edema as in any syndrome of congestive heart failure. Symptoms of angina pectoris are generally absent, although chest pain of an ischemic type does occur in some patients. The blood pressure may be normal or low, or even elevated in some patients.[10]

The physical findings are similar to those found in other forms of dilated cardiomyopathy, lateral displacement of the apical pulse, an S-3 and S-4 heart sound, systolic murmurs, elevated venous pressure, hepatomegaly, and edema. The EKG findings are also nonspecific, with atrial and ventricular arrhythmias, intraventricular conduction abnormalities, pathologic "Q" waves, and decreased QRS voltage as common findings. The chest X-ray generally shows a symmetric cardiomegaly, and cardiac catheterization reveals reduced output, high diastolic pressures, and pulmonary hypertension. The histologic features are varied and nonspecific; myocardial fiber hypertrophy and fibrosis as well as lipid or glycogen vacuolization are found.[11]

Alcoholic cardiomyopathy is not an inevitably fatal condition, and improvement frequently follows abstinence from alcohol, particularly in those patients in whom cardiac symptoms are of recent onset. It is likely that many of the cases of cardiomyopathy that receive heart transplantations have an alcoholic basis. This is important to note because continued drinking may contribute to a poor-outcome post-transplantation. All cases of cardiomyopathy should be evaluated for possible alcoholism.

Gastrointestinal System

Disturbances attributable to the gastrointestinal tract occur commonly following alcohol use, particularly, in higher and chronic administration. Any complaint arising from the gastrointestinal system deserves an evaluation of alcohol use and possible alcoholism. Alcohol produces irritation and inflammation of the mucosa lining the gastrointestinal tract. Frank ulceration may occur with chronic alcohol use.[12]

The well-known "heartburn" is due to esophageal reflux with esophagitis that commonly occurs with irritation and inflammation of the gastroesophageal junction by alcohol. Severe vomiting may result in mucosal tears at this junction, with hematemesis as in the Mallory–Weiss syndrome. Esophageal varices are an expression of portal hypertension from liver disease, also often induced by alcohol. These varices are engorged, dilated capillaries that represent a collateral circulation. Significant and sometimes fatal hemorrhage may occur from these varices.[13]

The stomach and duodenum are sites vulnerable to the corrosive effects of alcohol. Short- and long-term alcohol ingestion is associated with gastritis, erosive gastritis, gastric ulceration, atropic gastritis, and gastric hemorrhage. Furthermore, duodenitis and duodenal ulcerations are a direct result of chronic alcohol irritation and inflammation. Scarring and obstruction may result from chronic ulceration.[14]

Chronic administration of alcohol may result in chronic pancreatitis. However, acute ingestion of alcohol is associated with an alteration of the secretion of the pancreatic enzymes and abnormalities in intestinal absorption in acute and chronic alcohol use. Abdominal pain and vomiting are common during acute pancreatitis. The pain is poorly localized to the upper abdomen, radiating to the back. Other signs may be lacking in mild cases, and in more severe cases, hypoactive bowel sounds and rebound tenderness suggestive of peritonitis may be present. In cases of high fever, a pancreatic abscess may be suspected, also an abdominal mass, a pseudocyst, and shifting dullness, and ascites may be encountered. Helpful diagnostic features are serum amylase, a KUB, ultrasonography, and CT or MRI scanning.[15,16]

Diabetes mellitus or hyperglycemia is a complication resulting from the eventual destruction of the islet cells in the pancreas from persistent, alcohol-induced, chronic pancreatitis. Often insulin is necessary to compensate for the lost insulin production in the fibrosed, contracted pancreas. At times, replacement therapy of pancreatic enzymes for pancreatic insufficiency may be necessary.[17]

Malabsorption and diarrhea are common in alcoholics and are a result of a number of interactive factors. These include alterations in gastric motility, mucosal erosions, and impaired transport of glucose, amino acids, and vitamins, particularly thiamine and vitamin B12 and the minerals calcium and magnesium.[18]

The liver is a particularly vulnerable organ in alcohol consumption, in part because it is where alcohol is metabolized and broken down for reuse and elimination from the body. The most common manifestation is fatty metamorphosis or fatty liver. For some alcoholics, a fatty liver may precede the onset of alcoholic cirrhosis. However, a large number of those who consume alcohol will develop fat in the liver but not cirrhosis. In fact, evidence in animals suggests that fatty metamorphosis occurs regularly with acute ingestion of alcohol. Transient, mild elevations of liver enzymes, particularly ALT and AST, will occur. These return to normal within a few weeks.[19,20]

Alcoholic hepatitis is a severe condition that is characterized by jaundice, fever, anorexia, and right-upper-quadrant pain. The liver histologically shows parenchymal and portal infiltration with polymorphonuclear leukocytes, steatosis, cholestasis, and sometimes hyaline bodies. The serum levels of ALT, AST, and GDH are elevated, at times, at high levels. Prolongation of the prothrombin time and ascites may occur.[21]

Alcoholic cirrhosis is not a particularly common condition among alcoholics as a total population. However, its prevalence increases in older and more chronic populations of alcoholics. The overall prevalence rate for cirrhosis is 5% to 10% of all alcoholics. The most common signs of uncomplicated cirrhosis are weight loss, weakness, and anorexia. In more severe cases, the signs may include jaundice, a small or large liver, splenomegaly, ascites, asterixis, testicular atrophy, edema, spontaneous peritonitis, gynecomastia, spider angiomata, palmar eythema, and Dupuytren's contracture. Laboratory findings are hypoalbuminemia and hyperglobinemia, with or without elevation of liver enzymes. Cirrhosis is scarring of the liver from alcohol with a microscopic picture of fibrosis of portal and central zones and an overall distortion of the architecture of the liver, which may be small and shrunken.[22,23]

Serious complications from cirrhosis are ascites, esophageal varices, hepatroenal syndrome (renal failure) and hepatic encephalopathy, coma and death. Once cirrhosis has developed, the life expectancy is around 50% if abstinence is maintained and significantly less if alcohol is continued to be ingested. It is not known why and which individuals will develop cirrhosis except that it tends to occur in chronic, older drinkers—although there are many exceptions to this rule.[24,25]

Nutritional Complications

Alcohol and nutritional status are interrelated. Alcohol intake may interfere with the absorption, digestion, metabolism, and utilization of nutrients, particularly vitamins. The use of alcohol as a source of calories to the exclusion of other food sources, including nutrients, may also lead to a nutrient deficiency.[25,26]

Alcohol disrupts absorption of nutrients in the various ways outlined in previous sections by acting on the intestinal wall such as the small intestine and damaging organs such as the pancreas that are responsible for digestion. The effect of alcoholism on metabolism is to alter the inactivation and activation of the nutrients. For instance, alcohol decreases the net synthesis of pyridoxal phosphate from pyridoxine. These effects have been linked to the oxidation of ethanol and may involve the displacement and subsequent degradation of pyridoxal-5-phosphate from its cytosol-binding protein by phosphatase and results in a net decrease in activation. These nutritional effects of alcohol are more than an academic interest. Admission to hospitals for malnutrition for alcoholism remains a significant portion of admissions for malnutrition. Alcoholism is suggested as the most common cause of vitamin and trace-element deficiency in adults in the United States. And malnutrition remains a significant cause of admissions to general hospitals.[27,28]

The regular consumption of alcohol itself contributes to the poor intake of other food stuffs containing proper nutrients. Alcohol contains calories, supplying 7.1 kcal/g. Thus a consumer of 600 ml of 86-proof distilled spirits derives 1,500 kcal or more than one half of his or her daily caloric needs. The calories derived from alcohol are called "empty" calories because of the small amounts of vitamins, minerals, essential amino acids, or essential fatty acids contained in most alcoholic beverages. Primary malnutrition resulting from a decrease in the actual ingestion of nutrients is frequently associated with regular and heavy alcohol use.

1. *Folic acid deficiency.* Megaloblastic anemia is common in malnourished alcoholics and most often is due to folate deficiency. Thrombocytopenia and granulocytopenia may accompany the megaloblastic changes, especially if the folate level is severely low. The deficiency results from poor intake and disruption of absorption in the small bowel. The hematologic manifestations of the folate deficiency are rapidly reversible despite persistently low serum levels.[29,30]

2. *Pyridoxine deficiency.* Pyridoxine deficiency has been implicated in the development of sideroblastic anemias in the alcoholic. The sideroblastic changes induced by ethanol and a diet low in pyridoxine is reversed by the intake of the vitamin in spite of continued alcohol ingestion.[31]

3. *Thiamine deficiency.* The thiamine deficiency in the alcoholic may result from malabsorption and perhaps defective activation of thiamine. Thiamine deficiency is the cause

of Wernicke–Korsakoff syndrome. It is certain that latent or subclinical thiamine deficiency is common in the alcoholic, and the administration of parental glucose without thiamine may precipitate Wernicke's encephalopathy in such patients.[32]

4. *Iron deficiency.* Iron deficiency is usually only present when other factors related to iron deficiency are present such as gastrointestinal bleeding and infection. Iron overload or excess is more likely than deficiency because of increased iron absorption from a pancreatic insufficiency. Because an anemia from another cause may be present, iron may be given incorrectly.[33,34]

5. *Zinc deficiency.* Zinc deficiency may be associated with the pathogenesis of night blindness seen in alcoholics because of its role as a cofactor of vitamin A dehydrogenase, the enzyme responsible for the conversion of retinol to retinal.[35]

6. *Fat soluble vitamin deficiency.*

a. *Vitamin A.* A deficiency in vitamin A may result from a decreased uptake from malabsorption (steatorrhea), impaired storage, increased degradation, and diminished activation. Chronic consumption of ethanol decreases hepatic vitamin A levels. Clinically, vitamin A deficiency is related to abnormal dark adaptation and hypogonadism. Repletion of vitamin A and zinc may reverse these conditions but should be done cautiously because alcohol increases the hepatotoxicity of even moderate doses of vitamin A.[36,37]

b. *Vitamin D.* Vitamin D deficiency may result from decreased dietary intake, decreased absorption, and altered metabolism. Vitamin D depletion and impairment of calcium transport may lead to a decrease in bone density and increased susceptibility to fractures and asceptic necrosis.[38]

c. *Vitamin K.* Steatorrhea, decreased intake, and altered colonic microflora may combine to produce vitamin K deficiency. In patients with liver damage, further vitamin K deficiency may result in a depression of an already marginal synthesis of clotting factors and result in bleeding.[39]

Endocrinological Effects

Alcohol affects the endocrine system in a variety of ways by interacting at all levels of the endocrine axis. The levels at which alteration from alcohol may occur are the hypothalamus, the pituitary, adrenal, thyroid, and gonadal glands. Furthermore, liver injury from alcohol disturbs the peripheral metabolism of hormones by changes in hepatic blood flow, protein binding, enzymes, cofactors, or receptors.

1. *Adrenocortical function.* Chronic alcohol consumption results in increased plasma cortisol levels. Occasionally, alcohol use is associated with Cushingnoid changes that are increased plasma-cortisol levels more consistently, an abnormal response to dexamethasone, and evidence of pituitary dysfunction is present. Alcohol activates the hypothalamic–pituitary–adrenal axis to promote ACTH release and cortisol secretion.[40,41]

2. *Adrenomedullary function.* Alcohol consumption results in stimulation of adrenal medullary secretion of catecholamines. The peripheral metabolism of catecholamines shifts from an oxidative (3-methoxy-4-hydroxymandelic acid) to a reductive pathway (3-methoxy-4-hydroxyphenylglycol), a change that reflects an increase in the NADH/NAD ratio or acetaldehyde production. This ratio change may be important in the generation of condensation products in the formation of the tetrahydroisoguinolines.[42] Chronic alcohol consumption also leads to the stimulation of the secretion of catecholamines from the sympathetic portion of the autonomic nervous system. Alcohol withdrawal is characterized by alterations in vital signs and arousal state that are indicative of a massive release of catecholamines.

3. *Thyroid function.* Alcohol administration increases the liver to plasma ratios of thyroid hormone that may lead to a hepatic "hyperthyroidism." This state is responsible for increased oxygen consumption, local anoxia, and possibly liver injury.[43,44]

4. *Gonadal function.* Alcohol consumption decreases plasma testosterone, an effect that results from a decrease in production and increased metabolic clearance of the hormone. Alcoholic cirrhosis is known to lead to primary hypogonadism with subsequent feminization. The pathological basis is multifactorial—destruction of the testosterone-producing cells in the testes; elevated estradiol and estrone levels; and increased conversion of testosterone and androstenedione to estrogen because of decreased breakdown by the liver. The clinical manifestations are loss of male secondary sex characteristics and a feminization, including decreased libido, hair, muscle mass, gynecomastia, and smooth feminine skin. These changes may or may not be reversible, depending on the degree of permanent damage.[45,46]

5. *Pituitary function.* The release of the gonadotropin from the hypothalmic–pituitary axis is defective. Also, the release of the antidiuretic hormone in the posterior pituitary gland is inhibited by alcohol. The end result is a diuretic action of alcohol and subsequent dehydration from a lack of action of the antidiuretic hormone on the reabsorption of free water in the tubules in the kidney.[47]

6. *Alcoholic hypoglycemia.* This is due to an inhibition by alcohol of gluconeogenesis in the liver. Gluconeogenesis is the major source of glucose during chronic alcohol consumption particularly when other dietary sources of glucose are not available to the liver. The symptoms of hypoglycemia may be severe, with fatigue, tremors, seizures, and other manifestations of low blood sugar.

7. *Alcoholic ketosis.* This condition usually follows regular consumption of alcohol, anorexia, and hyperemesis. The level of beta-hydroxybutyrates are higher than that of acetoacetate.[48]

Nervous System

Neurologic complications from chronic alcohol consumption are numerous and occur in most chronic drinkers. The type and number of neurologic complications depend on the severity of the alcohol use, nutritional status, and individual susceptibililty to alcohol.

The most common abnormality is a decrease in intellectual functioning or dementia syndrome with a subsequent decrease in recent memory, abstractions, calculations, general knowledge, and other aspects of cognitive functions. Studies show that a reduction in IQ may result from as little as 2 ounces of alcohol consumed on a regular basis over a prolonged period of months. Studies of alcoholics show that the depression in IQ may be reversible, improving over a period of months and years from the time of cessation of alcohol use.[49,50]

Furthermore, CT scans (computerized tomography) of the brain have confirmed that cerebral atrophy occurs in alcoholics frequently at any age but is more commonly and pronounced at older ages. The changes seen in the CT scans are representative of a decrease in brain mass with a concomitant increase in ventricular size. The changes are diffuse and widespread, indicative of a generalized effect of alcohol in the brain. The cerebral atrophy correlates with impairments in the intellect. With abstinence, atrophy as well as the reduction in IQ is noted to reverse with subsequent CT scanning of the brain and retesting of the IQ.

The underlying mechanism is a direct toxicity by alcohol on the neurons and their processes, the axons, and dendrites as well as the supporting cells, the astroglia. These neuropathological changes have been noted in animal and human studies, when nutritional factors have been controlled for.[49]

Interestingly, the most classic neurological syndrome from chronic alcohol consumption may not be due to the direct toxic effects of alcohol. Wernicke–Korsakoff syndrome is the result of a thiamine deficiency but does not play a role in the direct toxicity on nerve cells. The neuropathological changes are due to alterations in the cerebellum, brain stem, and diencephalon. These changes are often small hemorrhages and infarct in the structures.[49]

The clinical manifestations are predictable for Wernicke's syndrome and include a delirium with a clouded sensorium and confusion, ophthalmoplegia, nystagmus, and ataxia. Peripheral neuropathies are commonly associated with the syndrome. All as aspects of the syndrome will improve with the administration of thiamine, although not always completely. Many of the patients with Wernicke's syndrome will develop the Korsakoff syndrome, although a few will return to their premorbid state. The Korsakoff syndrome is characterized by a profound loss in recent memory out of proportion to the other cognitive deficits. In other words, the Korsakoff patient may not remember dates and names but can calculate and abstract reasonably well in an intact personality.[49]

Alcoholic peripheral neuropathy is characterized by diminished sensitivity to touch, pinprick, and vibration objectively, and paraesthesias subjectively. These symptoms appear bilateral and symmetrical, most prominent in the distal portions of the extremities, in greater frequency and severity in the lower extremities. Both sensory and motor nerves are affected.[49]

The alcoholic myopathy can be acute, subacute, and chronic in onset. Muscle weakness and atrophy may be present. More often an elevated CPK (creatinine phosphokinase) occurs in association with the symptoms of muscle cramps, weakness, and occasional dark urine (myoglobinuria). In severe cases, the rhabdomyolysis produces significant myoglobinuria with renal failure that may be fatal. Most likely, the etiology of the muscle damage is the direct toxic effect of ethanol on muscle. In most cases, discontinuation of alcohol consumption leads to improvement of the myopathy.[1,2,49]

Cancer

Heavy drinking increases the risk of cancer in the tongue, mouth, oropharynx, hypopharynx, esophagus, larynx, and liver. In the United States, these sites represent approximately 10% of all cancers in the white population and 12% in the black population.

1. *Buccal cavity, pharynx, and larynx.* Cancers of the mouth, pharynx, and larynx appear to be related to heavy drinking. Tobacco is the leading risk factor for the development of these cancers, but alcohol carries an additional, increased risk to the development of cancer. Of course, cigarette smoking commonly occurs among alcoholics. One study showed that 93% of men and 91% of women in a group of alcoholic outpatients were smokers, proportions far above the prevalence for smoking in the general population. A study, however, separated out the individual risk for cancer of the mouth and concluded that "heavy drinkers" had a tenfold greater risk of having cancer of the mouth than minimal drinkers. As the amount of alcohol consumed is increased, the relative risk of cancer of the mouth, extrinsic larynx, and esophagus was also increased, much more so with whiskey than beer and wine.[51]

2. *Esophagus.* Two-thirds of patients with cancer of the esophagus also have a history of heavy alcohol use. Investigators have shown a relationship between heavy drinking, especially of whiskey or other spirits, and esophageal cancer, after corrections for age and tobacco were made. Smoking has been reported to be less important than alcohol in the absence of heavy drinking.

3. *Large intestine and rectum.* In studies, a strong asso-

ciation between rectal and colonic cancer and alcohol, particularly beer, exists.[52]

4. *Liver, primary.* Worldwide, almost 90% of all liver-cell cancer arises in cirrhotic organs. The typical person in whom a primary cancer of the liver (hepatoma) occurs is an alcoholic with cirrhosis. However, hepatoma may occur in alcoholics who do not have cirrhosis. The hepatoma seems to occur 2 to 8 years after the onset of cirrhosis.

5. *Pancreas.* There may be an association between alcohol consumption and pancreatic malignancy, particularly if pancreatitis exists before the onset of the pancreatic malignancy.

Infectious Diseases

Pneumonia is a frequent cause of illness and death for alcoholics. In some studies, as many as 50% of all patients admitted with pneumonia were alcoholics. Also, tuberculosis appears to be prevalent among alcoholics. Other infectious diseases that are overrepresented among alcoholics are bacterial meningitis, peritonitis, and ascending cholangitis. Less serious infections are chronic sinusitis, pharyngitis, and other minor infections.[1,2]

The basis for an increased risk for infection among alcoholics is a depressed immune system by alcohol at the various sites of the immune defense in the reticuloenthial system. Studies have demonstrated decreased white cell production and response in active drinkers, in addition to impaired antibody production.

References

1. Lieber CS: *Medical Disorders of Alcoholism.* Philadelphia, W. B. Saunders Co., 1982.
2. Petersdorf RG, Adams RD, Braunwald E, et al. eds.: *Harrison's*

Principles of Internal Medicine, 10th ed. New York, McGraw-Hill Publishers, 1983.

3. Miller NS, Gold MS, Cocores JA, Pottash AC: Alcohol dependence and medical consequences. *New York State Journal of Medicine,* 1988 (Sept.); 88:476–481.

4. Mendelson JH, Mello NK: *The Diagnosis and Treatment of Alcoholism,* 2nd ed. New York, McGraw-Hill Book Co., 1985.

5. Clark LT, Friedman HS: Hypertension associated with alcohol withdrawal: Assessment of mechanisms and complications. *Alcoholism* 1985; 9:125–130.

6. Kannel WB, Sorlie P: Hypertension in Frammingham. In Paul O ed.: *Epidemiology and Control of Hypertension.* New York, Station Intercontinental Medical Book Corp., 1974.

7. Klatsky AL, Friedman GD, Siegelaub AB, et al.: Alcohol consumption and blood pressure. Kaiser-Permanente Multiphasic Health Examination data. *New Eng J Med* 1977; 296:1194–1200.

8. Friedman HS, Geller SA, Lieber CS: The effect of alcohol on the heart, skeletal and smooth muscles. In Lieber CS, ed.: *Medical Disorders of Alcoholism—Pathogenesis and Treatment,* Philadelphia, W.B. Saunders Company, pp. 436–479.

9. Fuster V, Gersh BJ, Giulaina ER, Tajik AJ, Brandenburg RO, Frye RL: The natural history of idiopathic dilated cardiomyopathy. *American Journal of Cardiology* 1981; 47:525–531.

10. Demakis JG, Proskey A, Rahimtoola SH, Jamil M, Sutton GC, Rosen KM, Gunnar RM, Tobin JR, Jr.: The natural course of alcoholic cardiomyopathy. *Ann Int Med* 1974; 80:293–297.

11. Evans W: Alcoholic cardiomyopathy. *Am Heart J,* 1961; 61:556–567.

12. Williams RR, Horn JW: Association of cancer sites with tobacco and alcohol consumption and socioeconomic status of patients: Interview study from the third national cancer survey. *J Nat Cancer Inst,* 1977; 58:547.

13. Eckardt FF, Grace ND, Kantrowitz PA: Does lower esophageal sphincter incompetency contribute to esophageal variceal bleeding? *Gastroenterology* 1976; 71:185–189.

14. Cooke AR: Ethanol and gastric function. *Gastroenterology,* 1972; 62:501–502.

15. Bank S: Acute and chronic pancreatitis. In Dent, TL, ed.: *Pancreatic Disease; Diagnosis and Therapy,* New York, Grune & Stratton, Inc., pp. 167–188.

16. Sarles H: Chronic calcifying pancreatitis—Chronic alcohol pancreatitis. *Gastroenterology,* 1974; 66:604–616.
17. Strum WB, Spiro HM: Chronic pancreatitis. *Ann Int Med,* 1971; 74:264–277.
18. Arvanitakis C, Greenberger NJ: Diagnosis of pancreatic disease by a synthetic peptide. A new test of exocrine pancreatic function. *Lancet,* 1976; 1:663–666.
19. Van Waes L, Lieber CS: Early perivenular sclerosis in alcoholic fatty liver, an index of progressive liver injury. *Gastroenterology,* 1977a; 73:646–650.
20. Van Waes L, Lieber CS: Glutamate dehydrogenase, a reliable marker of liver cell necrosis in the alcoholic. *Br J Med,* 1977b; 2:1508–1510.
21. DeRitis F, Coltorti M, Giusti G: Serum-transaminase activities in liver disease. *Lancet* 1972; 1:685–687.
22. Ratnoff OD, Patek AJ, Jr.: Natural history of Laennec's cirrhosis of the liver. An analysis of 386 cases. *Medicine* (Baltimore). 1942; 21:207–268.
23. Popper H, Lieber CS: Histogenesis of alcoholic fibrosis and cirrhosis in the baboon. *Am J Path,* 1980; 98:695–716.
24. Powell WJ, Klatskin G: Duration of survival in patients with Laennec's cirrhosis. Influence of alcohol withdrawal and possible effects of recent changes in general management of the disease. *Am J Med,* 1968; 44:406–420.
25. Rubin E, Lieber CS: Alcohol-induced hepatic injury in nonalcoholic volunteers. *New Eng J Med,* 1968; 278:869–876.
26. Veitch RL, Lumeng L, Li TK: The effects of ethanol and acetaldehyde on vitamin B6 metabolism in liver. *Gastroenterology,* 1974; 66:868.
27. Veitch RL, Lumbeng L, Li TK: Vitamin B6 metabolism in chronic alcohol abuse: The effect of ethanol oxidation on hepatic pyridoxal 5' phosphate metabolism. *J Clin Invest,* 1925; 55:1026–1032.
28. Vlahcevic ZR, Buhac I, Farrar JT, Bell CC, Swell L: Bile acid metabolism of cholic acid metabolism. I. Kinetic aspects of cholic acid metabolism. *Gastroenterology,* 1971; 60:491–498.
29. Herbert V, Zalusky R, Davidson CS: Correlation of folate deficiency with alcoholism and associated macrocytosis, anemia and liver disease. *Ann Intern Med,* 1963; 58:977–988.
30. Hermos JA, Adams WH, Liu YK, Sullivan LW, Trier JS: Mucosa

of the small intestine in folate-deficient alcoholics. *Ann Intern Med*, 1972; 76:957–965.

31. Hines JD, Cowan DH: Studies on the pathogenesis of alcohol-induced sideroblastic bone-marrow abnormalities. *New Eng J Med*, 1970; 283:441–446.

32. Tomasulo PA, Kater RMH, Iber FL: Impairment of thiamine absorption in alcoholism. *Am J Clin Nutr*, 1968; 21:1340–1344.

33. Eichner ER, Buchanan B, Smith JW, Hillman RS: Variations in the hematologic and medical status of alcoholics. *Am J Med*, 1972; 263:35–42.

34. Charlton RW, Jacobs P, Seftel H, Bothwell TH: Effect of alcohol on iron absorption. *Br Med J*, 1964; 2:1427–1429.

35. Russell RM, Morrison SA, Smith FR, Oaks EV, Carney E: Vitamin A reversal of abnormal dark adaptation in cirrhosis. *Ann. Intern. Med.*, 1978; 88:622–626.

36. Sato M, Lieber CS: Hepatic vitamin A depletion after chronic ethanol consumption in baboons and rats. *J Nutr*, 1981; 111:2015–2023.

37. Leo MA, Lieber CS: Hepatic vitamin A depletion in alcoholic liver injury. *New Eng J Med*, 1982; 307:597–601.

38. Baran DT, Teitelbaum SL, Berfield MA, Parker G, Cruvant EM, Avoli LV: Effect on alcohol ingestion on bone and mineral metabolism in rats. *Am J Physiol*, 1980; 238:507–510.

39. Cederbaum AI, Lieber CS, Toth A, Beatty DS, Rubin E: Effects of ethanol and fat on the transport of reducing equivalents into rat liver mitochondria. *J Biol Chem*, 1973; 248:4977–4986.

40. Mendelson JH, Stein S: Serum cortisol levels in alcoholic and nonalcoholic subjects during experimentally induced alcohol intoxication. *Psychosomatic Med*, 1966; 28:616–626.

41. Mendelson JH, Ogata M, Mello NK: Adrenal function and alcoholism. I. Serum cortisol. *Psychomatic Med*. 1971; 33:145–157.

42. Davis VE, Brown H, Huff JA, Cashaw JL: Ethanol-induced alterations of norepinephrine metabolism in man. *J Lab Clin Med*, 1967; 69:787–799.

43. Bleecker M, Ford DH, Rhines RK: A comparison of 131-Itriiodothyronine accumulation and degradation in ethanol-treated and control rats. *Life Sci*, 1969; 8:267–275.

44. Bernstein J, Videla L, Israel Y: Hormonal influences in the development of the hypermetabolic state of the liver produced by chronic administration of ethanol. *J Pharmacol Exper Therap*, 1975; 192:583–591.

45. Mendelson JH, Ellingboe J, Mello NK, Kuehnle J: Effects of alcohol on plasma testosterone and luteinizing hormone levels. *Alcoholism: Clin Exp Res*, 1978; 2:255–258.
46. Bhalla VK, Chen CJ, Gnanprakasam MS: Effect of in vivo administration of human chorionic gonadotropin and ethanol on the process of testicular receptor depletion and replenishment. *Life Sci*, 1979; 24:1315–1324.
47. Linkola J, Ylikhari R, Fyhrquist F, Wallenius M: Plasma vasopressin in ethanol intoxication and hangover. *Acta Physiol Scand*, 1978; 104:180–187.
48. Feinkel N, Singer DL, Arky RA et al.: Alcohol hypoglycemia. I. Carbohydrate metabolism in patients with clinical alcohol hypoglycemia and the experimental reproduction of the syndrome with pure ethanol. *J Clin Invest*, 1963; 42:1112–1133
49. Adams RP, Victor M: *Principles of Neurology*, 3rd ed. New York, McGraw-Hill, 1985.
50. Parsons OA, Leber WR: The relationship between cognitive dysfunction and brain damage in alcoholics: Casual, interactive, or epiphenomenal. *Alcoholism*, 1981; 5:326–343.
51. Durr HK, Bode J Ch, Gieseking R, Haase R, vArnim I, Beckman B: Anderungen der exokrinen Funktion der Glandula parotis und des Patienten mit Leberzirrhose und chronischem Alkoholismus. *Verh Dtsch Ges Inn Med*, 1975; 81:1322.
52. Martini GA, Wienbeck M: Begunstigt Alkohol die Entstehung eines Barrett-Syndroms (Endobrachyosophagus). *Dtsch Med Wochenschr*, 1974; 99:434.

6

Tolerance and Dependence

Few minds wear out; more rust out.

CHRISTIAN N. BOVEE

The answer to alcoholism probably does not lie in the understanding of tolerance and dependence, although they may lead scientists closer to the mystery of addiction to alcohol. Alcoholism is not a unique condition except that the addiction is to alcohol and not drugs, food, money, or power. Tolerance and dependence are also not uniquely found in alcoholism. Tolerance and dependence are naturally occurring "adaptations" found in the use of many drugs, either those to which man becomes addicted or those that benefit man as medications for diseases and other behaviors, especially those that are associated with other addictions.[1,2]

Tolerance is defined as the need to increase the dose or the amount of alcohol or "thing" to maintain the same effect from alcohol or that "thing." Another way of stating tolerance is that the effect is diminished or lost at a particular dose or amount of drug or "thing." Tolerance represents an adaptation of the brain or body to the continuous presence of a foreign substance, such as alcohol. The adaptation occurs at the pharmacodynamic site where the receptor is located on the target organ. In the instance of alcohol, the brain is the site where the addiction to alcohol most logically would appear to occur.[3,4]

The brain and body must function as normally as possible, and homeostatic mechanisms operate to insure that the brain and body are within psychological and physiological boundaries of normal functioning. When alcohol is present in the brain, the cells are changed by it to produce observable behaviors and subjective experiences that are characteristic of intoxication. The brain "resists" this alcohol-induced change by adapting in various ways at different levels. The brain is operating at a new and adjusted set point in the presence of alcohol to offset the effects. The brain opposes the alcohol effect. The net result of the combination of alcohol and the brain is to remain as near normal as the limits of tolerance of the brain allows and the amount of alcohol that needs to be neutralized.[4-6]

Dependence is defined as the onset of signs and symptoms of withdrawal upon the cessation of the use of alcohol or "thing." Withdrawal is a set or spectrum of predictable and stereotypic signs and symptoms that represent a deadaptation to the presence of alcohol or "thing." Frequently, the best antidote for the signs and symptoms of withdrawal is the cause, or alcohol. The hair of the dog that bit you is another way of stating that the drug, in this case alcohol, that induced the dependence syndrome will suppress the withdrawal.[7-9]

The brain had adjusted itself to a different level of functioning in the presence of alcohol but when the alcohol is withdrawn, the brain is "out on the limb" in the adapted state. In this state, the functioning is not in the normal range without the inducement of alcohol and the observable signs and symptoms are characteristic of the brain and body's attempt to return themselves to the previous set point for normal functioning. Dependence is a deadaptation of the body to the absence of alcohol, and the deadaptation is expressed in the typical signs and symptoms of withdrawal.[1,3]

Tolerance and dependence are on a continuum. As the tolerance is increased, the severity of the dependence is also increased. If the tolerance to alcohol in someone is particularly striking and large, then the dependence syndrome will be severe and significant. This direct relationship is seen with other drugs. The short-acting barbiturates show a rapid onset of tolerance and also have a more severe withdrawal syndrome than the longer acting barbiturates. Alcohol is a relatively short-acting drug so that the withdrawal syndromes tend to be noticeable and severe.[4]

Tolerance

There are many types of tolerance to alcohol. Tolerance is separated into two major categories for convenience—pharmacokinetic and pharmacodynamic tolerance. *Pharmacokinetic tolerance* is the dispositional capacity of an individual to drink alcohol. The dispositional tolerance is determined by a variety of physiological parameters. These include absorption, distribution, and elimination of alcohol. *Pharmacodynamic tolerance* is tolerance that develops at the receptor site; in the case of alcohol, the cell membrane.

Innate and Acquired Tolerance

The tolerance with which an individual is born is called *innate tolerance*. Innate or inborn tolerance varies widely from individual to individual and according to ethnicity. Larger individuals as a rule have a large capacity for alcohol as shown by an ability to drink larger amounts of alcohol with less effect of intoxication. The reason is that the blood volume is greater for larger individuals so that the concentration of a given dose of alcohol is less. In other words, larger people have more body water to dilute the peak of the blood-alcohol level during absorption.[1,5]

Other examples of innate tolerance are Orientals and alcoholics, at least, those who are at high risk for the development of alcoholism. As many as 80% of Orientals have adverse responses to small amounts of alcohol. This adversive reaction runs in families and appears to be a genetically transferrable condition. The reaction consists of signs and symptoms of a severe hangover that include nausea, vomiting, lightheadedness, a red facial and truncal flush, palpitations, and sleepiness. As little as an ounce or less of wine will trigger this reaction. Because the reaction is genetically determined, it represents an innate intolerance to alcohol.[12,18]

Alcoholics and high-risk individuals have an increased, innate tolerance to alcohol. Innate tolerance to alcohol is tolerance that is present before alcohol has been consumed and is an inherited trait. Innate tolerance is to be differentiated from acquired tolerance that develops in the presence of and as a result of alcohol use. Alcoholics appear to have this enhanced tolerance early in their drinking history, often, at the start of alcohol drinking. High-risk individuals before becoming alcoholic also have this increased capacity to drink alcohol without as great an intoxicating effect that low-risk individuals have. The innate tolerance or an inborn capacity to drink alcohol may be a marker for alcoholism before the onset of alcoholism.[13,14]

Acquired tolerance begins with the use of alcohol. Acquired tolerance is sometimes divided into acute and chronic tolerance to distinguish between what happens after a single dose of alcohol and after continuous use of alcohol. Studies have shown that tolerance develops after one dose of alcohol. When tolerance is measured objectively and subjectively in nonalcoholics and plotted along the blood-alcohol curve, tolerance to alcohol is noted at a higher blood level on the descending limb of the curve as compared to the ascending limb. The tolerance that develops so rapidly is nonetheless the same as expressed after chronic or regular use of alcohol.[6]

Chronic tolerance to alcohol, although probably qualitatively not different from acute tolerance, takes more time to develop and is larger in capacity. How much larger may not be that significant for alcohol, especially when compared to the degree of tolerance that develops in opiate use. The minimum lethal dose of morphine is about 10 times higher in opiate addicts with tolerance than in users without tolerance to opiates. The lethal dose of ethanol (alcohol) is essentially the same for alcoholics with tolerance to alcohol as those without tolerance to alcohol.

The importance of tolerance is often exaggerated. As people drink more over days, months, and years, they gradually need to drink more to obtain the same effect. This is called *tolerance*. A seasoned alcoholic at the prime of his or her drinking capacity may be able to drink, at most, twice as much as a teetotaler of similar age and health. Compared with tolerance for morphine and nicotine, which can be manyfold, tolerance for alcohol is modest.

The reason for increased tolerance in alcoholics may be for more than the obvious reason that one can drink more with a greater capacity without suffering the toxic effects of overdose. Tolerance appears to correlate with the euphoric effects of alcohol; the greater tolerance to alcohol, the greater the euphoria. Euphoria is that elusive sensation of feeling "high" or a sense of well-being, that all is right with oneself and the world. Drugs of abuse and addiction have both effects but differ in the proportion of either feeling high or a sense of well-being. Alcohol gives the user more of the latter effect of well-being, whereas cocaine provides an intense euphoria. Actually, the amount of euphoria from alcohol is milder than many drugs of abuse and addiction, such as co-caine and heroin.

Alcohol may be a drug preferred by the higher intellect. Animal studies suggest that alcohol has low reinforcing properties. Most animals do not prefer alcohol over water and do not use alcohol to excess or at all, unless no other liquid is available. The animal's aversion to alcohol suggests that feeling good is not a critical reason for using alcohol. Furthermore, alcoholics tend to lose this tolerance over time after chronic consumption and with aging. The loss of toler-ance to alcohol probably is what is responsible for the de-crease in euphoria and sense of well-being that occur with alcoholic consumption of alcohol. The mystery of addiction to alcohol or alcoholism is why the alcoholic continues to drink after the loss of tolerance and subsequent euphoria or well-being. The advanced alcoholic usually drinks to the stage of sedation, bypassing any high. Feeling good is not a reason to avoid drinking by the alcoholic. The time course for the loss in tolerance may be months, more often, a few years.[15]

Pharmacokinetic Tolerance

The principal site of absorption of alcohol is through the small intestine, mainly the duodenum. After alcohol is in-gested, it passes down the esophagus to enter the stomach, which acts as a reservoir. The emptying time of the stomach determines how long the alcohol is retained before it passes down to the duodenum for absorption. Contrary to popular belief, only a small amount of alcohol is absorbed from the stomach. Anything that delays the time that alcohol remains in the stomach will prolong the absorption. Food, partic-ularly fatty food, certain drugs, and volume of liquid will slow the passage of alcohol out of the stomach.[10]

Also, the concentration of alcohol is important as too high and low percentages of alcohol will not be absorbed as will the optimal dilution. Absolute alcohol (100%) irritates and inflames the lining of the stomach and so impedes its own absorption, whereas a dilute concentration (less than 20%) will also not be absorbed as quickly. The optimum dilution is around 40% that happens to be the percentage concentrations of most liquors distilled for distribution. (The proof of alcohol is equal to twice the percentage so that 80-proof vodka is equal to 45% alcohol.)[11]

The euphoria that some drinkers seek is dependent on how fast and how high the blood level of alcohol is reached. The faster and higher the blood-alcohol peak, the greater the euphoria or high. Anything that slows the absorption or dilutes the concentration of alcohol will lower both the time it takes to reach and the height of the peak blood level of alcohol. Food and diluted mixed drinks will not get some as drunk as fast as an empty stomach and a moderately concentrated alcoholic beverage.

The distribution of alcohol is everywhere within the body. Alcohol is a polar molecule that is soluble in water, so it goes wherever water goes, and water is a constituent of all living cells in the body. Although alcohol does not mix well with fats, it is such a small molecule in comparison to the barriers to it that it enters sanctuaries that are closed to other larger molecules.[11]

Alcohol is eliminated chiefly by a metabolic breakdown in the liver. A series of enzymes is responsible for the alteration of ethanol into various forms that are excreted, used elsewhere in the body for energy, building blocks for protein, and storage. The enzyme, alcohol dehydrogenase, converts alcohol to acetaldehyde. Acetaldehyde is a noxious chemical that when injected into humans produces a violent, nauseating reaction that resembles a severe hangover. In fact, acetaldehyde is the best single explanation we have for the hangover. Acetaldehyde is further converted by the enzyme, acetaldehyde dehydrogenase, to acetic acid. Acetic acid has many facets that include carbohydrates, fats, proteins, carbon dioxide, and water.[5,11]

A small amount of alcohol is excreted unchanged in the lungs, urine, and sweat; this accounts for about 2% as 98% of the alcohol is metabolized by the liver. This form of tolerance does not account for the tolerance that develops to alcohol because the blood level remains the same as tolerance appears. If breakdown by the liver was responsible for tolerance, then the blood level would decrease as the alcohol was metabolized.[5,11]

Pharmacodynamic Tolerance

The mechanism that explains tolerance most economically and logically is at the receptor site where alcohol acts. Pharmacodynamic tolerance to alcohol is tolerance that develops at the receptor site, which is the cell membrane in the case of alcohol. Alcohol acts to disrupt cell membranes. Cell membranes are the outer covering of mammalian cells, analogous to the skin in the human body. The cell membrane is composed of "phospholipids" that contain long-chain fatty acids. These fatty acids point toward the center of the cell in an alignment with each other that provides for order in the membrane. The order of the membrane is important for normal functioning of the cell. Alcohol causes these fatty acids to move about in a more fluid or disorderly way.[16,17]

The cell resists the action of alcohol to cause disordering to maintain as normal order as possible under the influence of alcohol. What the cell membrane does is to increase its intrinsic order so as to reset the set of point of the membrane closer to the prealcohol order. In the presence of alcohol, the membrane order is near normal, and in the absence of alcohol, the membrane is more ordered. A more ordered membrane is more rigid because the fatty acids are more resistant to motion that is caused by alcohol. The tolerance to alcohol is correlated with these rigid membranes. The development of more rigid membranes is an example of pharmacodynamic tolerance.[19,20]

The red blood cells of alcoholics are actually more rigid than nonalcoholics, when membranes are tested for their degree of fluidity or order. It cannot be determined by these studies if the more rigid red blood cells in alcoholics represent innate or acquired pharmacodynamic tolerance. The hope is to develop a blood test that will measure the amount of tolerance to alcohol as a marker for alcoholism.[21]

Cross-Tolerance

Cross-tolerance between alcohol and other drugs is an interesting but predictable occurrence. What this means is that someone who is tolerant to alcohol will also be tolerant to those drugs that share cross-tolerance with alcohol. Barbiturates and benzodiazepines are two classes of sedative/hypnotics that have cross-tolerance with alcohol. A well-known example is that alcoholics frequently require higher doses of these drugs to obtain the desired effect. Also, benzodiazepines such as librium, valium, and ativan are used to detoxify alcoholics during withdrawal. Because of the cross-tolerance, the signs and symptoms of alcohol withdrawal are suppressed by librium. Librium can also be used to suppress the signs and symptoms of withdrawal from barbiturates, such as secobarbital and pentobarbital.[16]

Dependence and Withdrawal

Dependence is a term that has undergone a lot of change in meaning as applied to alcohol and drugs. The term *dependence* has many meanings and derivations to professionals and nonprofessionals. The pharmacological definition of dependence is the onset of withdrawal on the cessation of the drug or alcohol. The pharmacological definition is the same as "physical dependence." Withdrawal is characterized by a predictable and stereotypical set of signs and symptoms that are typical for alcohol or a given drug. Withdrawal is a deadaptation of the brain and body to the absence of alcohol after a period of adaptation during the development of tolerance.

The signs and symptoms of the withdrawal of various drugs have some commonality and uniqueness. Withdrawal is a hyperexcitable state in response to the depressant action of alcohol. The sympathetic nervous system is discharging in withdrawal from many drugs, particularly, alcohol. The sympathetic nervous system is responsible for anxiety, apprehension, tremors, palpitations, sweating, irritability, high blood pressure, and other manifestations of an excited state. Anxiety and depression are common to the withdrawal of many drugs, including alcohol. As is evident, withdrawal is an unpleasant state that has negative feelings and significant medical consequences.[1,3]

Alcohol withdrawal should be considered as a spectrum of signs and symptoms of the abstinence state. At one end of the spectrum is anxiety, tremors, palpitations, and hypertension, whereas the more severe part of the spectrum consists of seizures, delusions, hallucinations, delirium tremens, and death. Delirium tremens, untreated, has a mortality rate of 50%. DTs constitute a confused and cloudy sensorium with disorientation to time and place, hypervigilant and agitated state, marked tremors of extremities and body, significant elevations of blood pressure and pulse, terrifying visual hallucinations, usually, of animals, that is, snakes, severe dehydration from hypermetabolic state, and prostration. The causes of death in DTs is from self-inflicted injury as a result of the confusion and hallucinations, heart failure from arrhythmias, and pneumonias. With proper treatment the mortality and morbidity can be reduced to less than 25%.[1,3]

Other features of the abstinence syndrome or spectrum are auditory hallucinations or hearing voices in the absence of a source, visual hallucinations, again, animals such as bugs or worms, and paranoid delusions that someone is out to harm them in the absence of harm toward them. The abstinence syndrome can mimic other known psychiatric conditions such as anxiety disorders, manic–depression, schizophrenia, phobias, and obsessive–compulsive disorders.

The dependence syndrome in its milder forms develops after a small dose of alcohol in a nondrinker. Fluctuations in mood, blood pressure and pulse, and disturbances in sleep and appetite can occur after only a few ounces of alcohol. It is a myth that high doses of alcohol over prolonged periods of time are necessary to develop "physical dependence." The hangover is an example of alcohol withdrawal or a dependence syndrome. The hangover results in response to the cessation of the use of alcohol and is characterized by anxiety, depression, headache, malaise, and elevated blood pressure and pulse. Furthermore, the more severe signs of withdrawal that include seizures and DTs can develop only after a few weeks of regular alcohol use in susceptible individuals.

The essential features of alcohol withdrawal and a suggested detoxification schedule are presented in Tables 1, 2, and 3.

References

1. Jaffe JH: Drug addiction and drug abuse. In Gilman AG, Goodman LS, Rall TW, Murad F. eds: *The Pharmocological Basis of Therapeutics,* 7th ed., pp. 532–581. New York, Macmillan, 1985.
2. Miller NS, Dackis CA, Gold MS: The relationship of addiction, tolerance and dependence to alcohol and drugs: A neurochemical approach. *Journal of Substance Abuse and Treatment,* 1987; 4:197–207.
3. Victor M, Adams RP: The effect of alcohol on the nervous system. *Research Publications, Association for Research in Nervous and Mental Disease,* 1953; 32:526–573.
4. Hill MA, Bangham AD: General depressant drug dependency:

TABLE 1. Alcohol Intoxication

Signs

Smell of alcohol on breath
Incoordination
Slurred speech
Vertigo
Vomiting
Tremors
Unconsciousness
Unsteady gait

Symptoms

Slowed thinking
Decreased self-control
Decrease muscular control
Euphoria or depression
Impaired memory for recent events
Labile emotion with weeping or laughter
Exaggeration of underlying personality traits
Self- and other-directed violence
Emergence of repressed and suppressed desires
Irritability
Loquacity
Failure to meet responsibilities
Amnesia (blackouts)

A biophysical hypothesis. *Advances in Experimental Medicine and Biology,* 1975; 59:1–9.

5. Majchrowicz E, Noble EP: *Biochemistry and Pharmacology of Ethanol,* Vol. 1. New York: Plenum Press, 1979.
6. Wilson JR, Erwin G, McClearn GE, Plomin R, Johnson RC, Ahern FM, Cole RE: Effects of behavior: II. Behavioral sensitivity and acute behavioral tolerance. *Alcoholism,* 1984; 8:4.
7. Goldstein DB: The effects of drugs on membrane fluidity. In Cowan WM, Shooter EM, Stevens CF, Thompson RC, eds.: *Annual Review of Pharmacology,* 1984; 24:43–64.

TABLE 2. Alcohol Withdrawal (Peak Period 1–4 days)

Signs

Hand tremor
Diaphoresis
Tachycardia and elevated blood pressure
Dilated pupils
Increase in temperature
Seizures
Restlessness
Hyperactivity, agitation
Ataxia
Clouding of consciousness

Symptoms

Anxiety and panic attacks
Paranoid delusions or ideation
Illusions
Disorientation
Hallucinations, either of rapidly moving small animals such as snakes or Lilliputian hallucinations (auditory hallucinations are rare)

8. Jellinek EM: The disease concept of alcoholism. New Brunswick, NJ, Hillhouse Press, 1960.
9. Edwards G, Auf A, Hodgson R: Nomenclature and classification of drug and alcohol-related problems: A WHO memorandum. *Ball Who*, 1981; 59:225–242.
10. Lieber CS: *Medical Disorders of Alcoholism Pathogenesis and Treatment.* Philadelphia, W.B. Saunders Company, 1982.
11. Melium KL, Morrelli HF: *Clinical Pharmacology,* 2 ed., New York, Macmillan, 1978.
12. Miller NS, Goodwin DW, Jones FC, Anand MM, Pardo MP, Gabrielli WF, Pottash AC, Gold MS: Antihistamine blockade of alcohol-induced flushing in Orientals. *Journal of Studies on Alcohol*, vol. 49(1), January, 1988:16–20.
13. Goodwin DW: Alcoholism and heredity. *Archives of General Psychiatry*, 1979; 36:57–61.

TABLE 3. Alcohol Detoxification

Mild Withdrawal

Librium: 25–50 mg po every 4 hours prn for

    systolic blood pressure>150
    diastolic blood pressure>90
    pulse>100
    T>101
    tremulousness

Librium: 25–50 mg po prn for insomnia ×2 days.

Moderate Withdrawal

Librium: 25–50 mg po qid day 1
             20–40 mg po qid day 2
             10–30 mg po qid day 3

    (optional)

    20 mg po qid day 4
    10 mg po qid day 5

    May need to adjust based on signs and symptoms of alcohol withdrawal

Severe Withdrawal

Librium: 25–50 mg po every hour while awake (to sedate)

    systolic blood pressure>150
    diastolic blood pressure>90
    pulse>100
    temp>101
    tremulousness

---

14. Goodwin DW: Alcoholism and genetics. *Archives of General Psychiatry*, 1985; 42:171–174.
15. Tabakoff B, Ritzmann RF, Raju TS, Deitrich RA: Characterization of acute and chronic tolerance in mice selected for inherent differences in sensitivity to ethanol. *Alcoholism: Clinical and Experimental Research*, 1980; 4:70–73.

16. Goldstein DB: The effects of drugs on membrane fluidity. *Annual Review of Pharmacology and Toxicology,* 1984; 24:43–64.
17. Chin JH, Goldstein DB: Drug tolerance in biomembranes: A spin label study of the effects of ethanol. *Science,* 1977b; 196:684–685.
18. Chan AW: Racial differences in alcohol sensitivity. *Alcohol and Alcoholism,* 1986; 21:193–204.
19. Chin JH, Parsons LM, Goldstein DB: Increased cholesterol content of erythrocyte and brain membranes in ethanol tolerant mice. *Biochima et Piophysica Acta,* 1978; J13:358–363.
20. Chin JH, Goldstein DB: Membrane disordering action of ethanol: Variation with membrane cholesterol content and depth of the spin label probe. *Mol Pharmacol,* 1981; 19:425–531.
21. Miller NS: A blood marker for pharmacodynamic tolerance to alcohol. *Journal of Substance Abuse Treatment,* 1987; 4:93–102.

7

Clinical Diagnosis of Alcoholism

The trouble with doctors, I find, is that they seldom
admit that anything stumps them.

GEORGE JEAN NATHAN

Historical Perspective

The history of alcoholism is as old as prostitution. References are contained in the bible to the afflictions of those who are obsessed with wine or are possessed by demons who drive those to drink. The association of alcoholism with morality is ancient and remains a potent philosophy even today. Although alcoholism begins as a physical illness, a moral dilemma develops for most of those who suffer from it. Alcoholism is in many ways a paradox that mystifies those who have it and those who study and treat it. Because morality is such a prevalent part of the disease and its treatment, the diagnosis of alcoholism is difficult for the modern-day physician to grasp intuitively and apply the principles objectively.

The mind itself has been subjected to the test of morality throughout the history of medicine. Mental illness is a new concept developed in the twentieth century. Only a few decades ago schizophrenia and other psychiatric disorders were a product of the influence of the devil on the psyche. The disorders are readily accepted by many, although not all, as expressions of a physical or biochemical abnormality in the brain that controls and consumes the spirit and mental life of the individual. The Greeks espoused that some subversive spirit was the etiologic agent in the condition called hysteria. The treatments were aimed at controlling and ridding the individual of the spirit.

A popular diagnosis in the late nineteenth century was "moral inebriate." This is, in fact, an accurate description of an alcoholic but not complete. Because moral problems are a consequence of the alcoholism and do not cause it, it is a misleading choice of terminology. An example in medicine is the method for diagnosing syphilis before modern microbiological techniques unraveled the mystery of that disease. Syphilis was treated as a moral disease because those who tended to contract it were in the business of immorality, namely prostitutes. The treatment for syphilis was religious redemption or condemnation, depending on who was administering the treatment. Eventually it was discovered that a microbial agent, the spirochete, was the cause of all the myriad of manifestations of syphilis. The treatment then became penicillin. Because penicillin is effective only in the earlier stages of syphilis, early diagnosis is stressed.

In the early 1900s, a Yale doctor developed a most important concept that has revolutionized the diagnosis and treatment of alcoholism of mostly nonphysicians. Dr. E. M. Jellinek formulated the "disease concept of alcoholism" that is not yet accepted by most practicing physicians. Although the American Medical Association issued a formal statement in 1951 that declared that alcoholism was a "treatable" disease, the debate over that statement is very much alive today in medical communities.

The debate over the disease concept is critically important because whether or not the physician concerns himself or herself with the diagnosis or not depends on whether alcoholism is a disease. If it is not a disease, then the physician is not inclined to make it a part of his or her medical practice, viewing it rather as domain of other professionals or the alcoholic. Probably one of the reasons medical schools do not offer much in the curriculum regarding alcoholism is that alcoholism has not been considered a medical disease.

The underlying abnormality that is fundamental to the disease of alcoholism is relatively easy to define, namely loss of control over the chemical alcohol. All definitions of alcoholism ultimately rest on this observation. The alcoholic has lost the ability (or never possessed it) to control the use of alcohol and to avoid even the acquisition of alcohol. From the phenomena of loss of control is derived most of the sensible definitions of alcoholism and the identifiable manifestations of alcoholism. The etiology of the loss of control is neurochemical in origin, being based in the brain, and translated into mental and behavioral reality. Alcohol as a chemical interacts with the neuronal substrate to produce the predictable and stereotypic loss of control over alcohol inherent to alcoholism.

Great strides were made when alcoholism began to be considered a primary disorder. One of the major impediments to the diagnosis and treatment of alcoholism has been the attribution of alcoholism or the reasons for drinking to another, causal condition. The self-medication concept arose from the psychoanalytic theory that is based on psychic determinism. Psychic determinism is a useful concept that states that psychic events are caused by one another, particularly, early life experiences lead to and "determine" later feelings and thinking. When the reality of the moment is not congruent with the memories of the reality of the past, a conflict arises that is disharmonious to the ego. Other distressing conflicts arise from the collision of the passionate desires of the id with the ego and the punitive superego with the ego. The ego in desperation reaches for and is relieved by alcohol. Alcohol acts as an anesthetic to numb the harsh and unpleasant feelings that are plaguing the ego.

Biological psychiatry adheres to a similar construct of self-medication, only it differs in theoretical interpretations. Important and pathological symptoms by their injurious and noxious effects lead to alcohol use for amelioration. The symptoms of anxiety, depression, hallucinations, and delusions that are distressing to the possessor are treated with alcohol. The alcohol is used to medicate these pathological states that are underlying as causative agents. Alcohol use is only an attempt to treat an already existing abnormality.

The assumption in both regards is that alcohol is pleasant and relieves these unpleasant conditions. What adds to the credibility is that the common or laymen's way of thinking about alcohol use and alcoholism is very similar. The argument for self-medication as the etiology of alcoholism is similar to Plato's argument for the existence of God, which is that God exists because most people think He does. Although Plato's argument may be true, the self-medication concept probably has only minor validity in the origin of alcoholism. Once alcoholism begins, the consequences of drinking far outweigh any therapeutic effects so that the ratio of benefit to liability is reversed. Alcoholism is the mysterious condition whereby the use of alcohol continues without apparent reward and in spite of severe adverse consequences produced by the alcoholism.

The diagnosis of alcoholism advanced greatly when alcoholism was given the antecedent position instead of the consequent position. Jellinek introduced the notion that alcoholism caused a variety of manifestations that are consequent to loss of control over the use of alcohol. Useful schemes for diagnosing alcoholism were developed that emphasized the consequences of alcoholism. The National Council on Alcoholism and other authoritative groups developed criteria for alcoholism that required identification of psychological, physical, and sociological impairments from abnormal alcohol use. Although these criteria are useful and do identify a substantial number of alcoholics, the consequences do not describe the essential features of alcoholism.

Problems also arise from disagreement as to what is a consequence and what is its relevance. For instance, physicians tend to rely heavily on medical consequences that are not present in the majority of alcoholics. Furthermore, the consequences are frequently denied by the alcoholic so that ascertainment of the consequences is often elusive and difficult. Also consequences may result from alcohol use in those who are not alcoholic, that is, younger drinkers tend to drink heavily and with some consequences but are not always alcoholic. Finally, the consequences of alcoholism are attributed to other conditions, or, sometimes, back to the consequences. An alcoholic may have marital or employment problems because of the alcoholism, but the reverse is sometimes asserted, that the bad marriage or boring job are causing the alcoholism, which does not happen.

The Concept of Addiction

The concepts of the behaviors that underlie and generate alcoholism are embodied in the concept of addiction. *Addiction* is a behavioral term that describes the behaviors that define the specific nature of the loss of control in regards to alcoholism. Addiction comprises only the bare minimum of alcoholism but is useful in identifying alcoholism and distinguishing it from other disorders (Table 4). Addiction is defined by three principle behaviors—preoccupation, compulsivity, and relapse. Addiction to alcohol is characterized

TABLE 4. Criteria for Abuse, Addiction, Tolerance, and Dependence

Abuse

1. Use outside the accepted norm
2. Abnormal use
3. Not addiction

Addiction

1. Preoccupation with acquisition of alcohol/drugs
2. Compulsive use in spite of adverse consequences
3. Recurrent pattern of use/relapse

Tolerance
1. Need to increase dose of drug to achieve same effect
2. Loss of effect from drug at a particular dose

Dependence

1. Stereotypic set of signs and symptoms or cessation of use of drug
2. Drug will abort its withdrawal symptoms

by the preoccupation with the acquisition of alcohol and the compulsive use and relapse to alcohol in spite of adverse consequences.

Preoccupation with alcohol is demonstrated in the acquisition of alcohol. The alcoholic is obsessed with alcohol. Alcohol has a high priority in the alcoholic's life to the exclusion of other important and vital needs. The alcoholic may neglect his or her basic needs such as self-care, health, and interpersonal relationships among family, employment, and other arenas of his or her life. The alcoholic may provide countless reasons why he or she is drinking, but the addiction to alcohol is major and preeminent. The alcoholic continues to be preoccupied with alcohol when sanity would forget it.

The compulsive use of alcohol is demonstrated by the

continued use of alcohol in spite of adverse consequences. The use of alcohol may or may not be regular. Compulsivity is marked by relentless and persistent use when common sense would dictate stopping and desisting from the use of alcohol. The consequences may be trivial or enormous, often, the latter without significant effect on curbing or eliminating the use of alcohol. The order of the cause and effect is critical. The cause of the adverse consequences is alcoholism, and not the reverse, that the adverse consequences lead to alcoholism.

Relapse is the sine qua non of alcoholism. Occasionally preoccupation with acquisition is, for some other reason than alcohol addiction, transient. Moreover, compulsive use may be temporary and precipitated by some event or condition. However, the pattern or recurrent use of alcohol in spite of adverse consequences is confirmatory of an addiction. The repeated return to the use of alcohol when common sense dictates moderation or abstinence is explained only by an addiction to alcohol. Relapse may be frequent and only after a few days of abstinence or after a prolonged period of years. An inability to cut back or reduce the alcohol intake is also considered relapse as it is indicative of loss of control over alcohol use.

Loss of control is pervasive to the three criteria of addiction. Behind preoccupation with acquisition, compulsive use, and relapse is loss of control of alcohol. Loss of control is relative and rarely (if even possible) absolute. Alcoholics can and do exert some control over alcohol use but always identifiable is a significant degree of loss of control. The loss of control is manifested differently for each alcoholic as drinking patterns vary, and consequences vary from individual to individual.

The consequences of the addiction to alcohol are what arouses suspicion of the diagnosis of alcoholism initially. The major life areas are the most easily detected and the most commonly affected, although any aspect of the individual may be affected by the alcohol addiction. The fundamental defect in alcoholism is a disturbance in interpersonal relationships between the alcoholic and others. This disturbance is manifested in interpersonal relationships with spouses, friends, employees and employers, the laws and society. A multitude of impairments are possible in any facet of the alcoholic's life.

Just as with loss of control, the impairments are relative and difficult to detect. Also, rationalizations and minimization of the consequences as well as misattribution are obstacles to the correct assessment of alcoholism as being responsible. Marital difficulties arise for a variety of reasons of which alcoholism is one cause, albeit, common. Job performance may be significantly affected before impairment is noticed. Employment is not a sensitive indicator of alcoholism as noticeable impairment of work performance is a late occurrence. Denial by the alcoholic and others frequently inhibits an accurate assessment of the consequences of alcoholism. The tendency is to look for other excuses than the drinking to explain the problems. The defenses are always working to distract the focus away from the alcoholism as the primary instigator.

Valid criteria available are contained in the *Diagnostic and Statistical Manual* which is published by the American Psychiatric Association. The manual is updated periodically and the current version is available as DSM-III-R (the revised third edition). The DSM-III-R is an attempt at formulating the essentials of alcoholism for clinical use. The criteria are operational so they can be applied to clinical conditions. The criteria have been validated in field trials and have been shown to be reliable indicators of an addiction to alcoholism.

What about tolerance and dependence? Tolerance and dependence are misleading clinical criteria to use in clinical practice. The relationship between tolerance and dependence is not direct as it is considered to be and is not bilateral as many think. Furthermore, tolerance and dependence are not specific to addiction. Although tolerance and dependence occur frequently in addiction, their low threshold for detection make them unreliable in clinical practice. Obtaining a history of tolerance and dependence in alcoholism where denial is an inherent part of the disease is formidable. Moreover, the development of tolerance and dependence is not often clinically significant in younger alcoholics who do not have a long history of chronic alcohol consumption. Only a minority of alcoholics demonstrate dramatic escalations in tolerance and withdrawal syndromes that include tremor, seizures, and delirium. The degree of tolerance and dependence to alcohol is mild compared to opiates, so that the criteria used for withdrawal are important determinants of whether dependence exists or not.

In general, physiological findings and serious medical complications are not particularly common in the modern, youthful alcoholic, although they are present in a substantial minority. The majority of the somatic complaints are minor. These tend to cluster in the cardiovascular, gastrointestinal, pulmonary, endocrinologic, and traumatic complications. Examples are transient, mild hypertension and tachycardia, esophagitis or heartburn, chronic, productive cough, menstrual and weight abnormalities, and bruises. It is imperative that the physician look beyond the "physical aspect" of the alcoholism at some of the psychological manifestations.

Some of the frequent psychological consequences of alcoholism are anxiety, depression, phobias, and suicidal thinking and less frequent, delusions, hallucinations, and suicidal actions. These psychological manifestations are usually transient in the acute phase but persist less intensely over a protracted period of months. These effects are secondary to the pharmacological properties of alcohol and the emotional changes that occur without the presence of alcohol.

The diagnosis of alcoholism can be made simply and effectively. Alcoholism is an insidious disorder that is cunning, baffling, and powerful to those who have it and those who must diagnose it. Alcoholism should be suspected when a major life problem or psychological, physical health condition exists in the setting of drinking. The diagnosis of an addiction to alcohol is confirmed by identifying a preoccupation with the acquisition of alcohol, compulsive use of alcohol, and a pattern of relapse or inability to reduce the use of alcohol in spite of adverse consequences.

Denial and rationalization are nearly always obstacles to obtaining an accurate history to make the diagnosis. Corroborative sources for history are often needed to obtain the necessary information to make the diagnosis. Family, employers, and others are potential sources of historical data. A high index of suspicion is necessary to make the diagnosis of alcoholism. Alcoholism is a common disorder that warrants the vigilance of the physician. Alcoholism masquerades as many other conditions, so the "atypical" cases of anything should prompt consideration of alcoholism.

Finally, alcoholism is a medical disease or disorder that is the responsibility of the physician and the medical profession. Doctors see more alcoholics than any other single contact than perhaps the legal system. Early diagnosis is critical and saves morbidity and mortality from alcoholism. Early diagnosis and intervention are possible and desirable. Making the diagnosis of alcoholism is not an intrusion into the life of the alcoholic but a saving of one's life. Making the diagnosis of alcoholism is a major and necessary step in solving health problems. Without a proper diagnosis, specific treatment for alcoholism cannot be instituted. The natural history of alcoholism is a chronic relapsing disorder that requires diagnosis and intervention for its arrestment.

Bibliography

1. Adams RP, Victor M: *Principles of Neurology. Third Edition.* New York, NY, McGraw-Hill, 1985.
2. *Alcoholics Anonymous. Third Edition.* New York, NY, Alcoholics Anonymous World Services, Inc., 1976.
3. Clark LT, Friedman HS: Hypertension associated with alcohol withdrawal: Assessment of mechanisms and complications of alcoholism. *Clin and Exp Research* 9:125–132, 1985.
4. Galizio M, Maisto SA: *Determinants of Substance Abuse.* New York, NY, Plenum Press, 1985.
5. Goodwin DW: Alcoholism and genetics. *Arch Gen Psychiatry* 42:171–174, 1985.
6. Goodwin DW: Familial alcoholism: A review. *J Clin Psychiatry* 45:14–17, 1984.
7. Goodwin DW, Guze SB: *Psychiatric Diagnosis. Third Edition.* London, Oxford University Press, 1984.
8. *Harrison's Principles of Internal Medicine. 10th Edition.* New York, NY, McGraw-Hill, 1983.
9. Hoffman FG: *A Handbook on Drug and Alcohol Abuse. Second Edition.* London, Oxford University Press, 1983.
10. Holden C: Alcoholism and the medical cost crunch. *Science* 235:1132, 1987.
11. Jaffe JH: Drug and addiction abuse, in Gilman AG, Goodman LS, Rall TW, Murad F (eds), *The Pharmacological Bases of Therapeutics. Seventh Edition.* New York, NY, Macmillan Publishing Co., 1985, pp. 532–581.
12. Lieber CS: *Medical Disorders of Alcoholism.* Philadelphia, PA, W.B. Saunders Co., 1982.
13. Mayfield DG: Alcohol and affect: Experimental studies, in Goodwin DW, Erickson CK (eds), *Alcoholism and Affective Disorders.* New York, SP Medical and Scientific Books, 1979, pp. 99–107.
14. Mendelson JH, Mello NK: *The Diagnosis and Treatment of Alcoholism. Second Edition.* New York, NY, McGraw-Hill, 1985.
15. Parsons, OA, Leber WR: The relationship between cognitive dysfunction and brain damage in alcoholics: Causal or epiphenomena. *Clin Exp Research* 5:326–343, 1981.
16. Schuckit MA: Alcohol patients with secondary depression. *Am J Psychiatry* 140:711–714, 1983.

17. Schuckit MA: Alcoholism and affective disorder: Diagnostic confusion, in Goodwin DW, Erickson CK (eds), *Alcoholism and Affective Disorders.* New York, SP Medical and Scientific Books, 1979, pp. 9–19.
18. Schuckit MA: The disease alcoholism. *Postgraduate Medicine* 64:78–84, 1978.
19. Vaillant GE: *The National History of Alcoholism.* Cambridge, MA, Harvard University Press, 1983.

8

Laboratory Diagnosis of Alcoholism and Drug Addiction

The Use of the Laboratory in the Diagnosis of Alcoholism and Drug Addiction

There are no laboratory markers or histopathological findings that are specific for alcoholism. The need for greater sensitivity and specificity in the laboratory diagnosis of alcoholism continues to exist. There are sensitive and specific tests available to detect the presence of alcohol and drugs. However, these tests only confirm the use of the drugs; the syndromes of alcoholism and drug addiction must be confirmed by clinical investigation.[1,2]

The laboratory markers available for the indirect measurement of alcohol use are many and have some clinical utility in diagnosis and treatment. These laboratory abnormalities

95

are associated with excessive alcohol consumption.[3,4] Unfortunately, these abnormalities exist in a variety of other conditions and are not specific for alcoholism. Furthermore, the abnormalities only detect active or recent drinking and often are not present in the typical intervening periods of abstinence, particularly in the early phases of alcoholism.[5,6]

The conventional laboratory markers are derived from the effects of alcohol on the liver enzymes, blood cells, serum lipids, immunoglobulins, and other blood chemistries. Although one value is not specific for recent effects of alcohol, the combination may produce a pattern that is highly suggestive of an alcohol effect. The confirmation of the diagnosis of alcoholism still rests with establishing the clinical criteria.[7]

Liver Enzymes

Gamma-glutamyltransferase (GGT) is the most commonly used laboratory marker of heavy drinking and alcoholism. In many studies, serum GGT is elevated in 75% to 80% of alcoholics and heavy drinkers. In a random sample of Swedish middle-aged males, 16% had an elevated serum GGT, 75% of which was related to alcohol ingestion.[8]

GGT plasma level correlates purely with the total amount of alcohol consumed and is not affected as much by the acuteness of the alcohol ingestion. Although it correlated somewhat with the period of time of excessive alcohol consumption, it may take 2 weeks for the serum GGT level to increase following alcohol use. During abstinence, the GGT returns to normal over 4 to 5 weeks or longer. The levels obtained are ordinarily in the low range and not high as in severe obstructive states and hepatocellular toxicity.

As indicated, the major drawback with this marker is nonspecificity. GGT is a membrane-bound enzyme in the sinusoids of the liver as well as in membranes surrounding larger bile ducts. For these reasons, plasma GGT is elevated in all diseases of the liver that involve the biliary system. Moreover, some drugs will increase GGT levels.[12]

Other liver enzymes that are indicative of liver injury are aspartate aminotransferase (ASAT) and alanine aminotransferase (ALAT). Both are nonspecific markers of alcohol consumption. However, arguments have been forwarded for greater specificity indicative of alcohol consumption if the ratio of ASAT to ALAT is greater than 2. Of importance is that an elevation in any of the liver enzymes does not mean or confirm irreversible or serious or impending liver damage. It only indicates an effect of alcohol on the liver cells. Other corroborative laboratory markers must be employed to distinguish the presence and extent of liver damage, that is, albumin, total proteins. Some studies show that these liver enzymes may be increased after as little as 1 ounce of 80-proof liquor.[10]

For all the liver enzymes, the conditions in addition to alcohol that may raise their level in the plasma, are the following: Liver diseases, liver-microsomal-system-inducing drugs (antiepileptics, anticoagulants, and barbiturates), obesity, diabetes, pancreatitis, heart failure, acute renal failure, severe trauma, high carbohydrate diet, Type IV hyperlipidemia, increased age, smoking, pregnancy, and gender (males exhibit higher levels).[9]

MCV Mean Corpuscular Volume (MCV)

The hematological system is another important and reliable, although nonspecific, measurement of chronic alcohol intake. An increase in the mean corpuscular volume (MCV) is found in 31% to 96% of alcoholic patients. As with liver enzymes, the MCV is increased by other things, such as vitamin B12 and folic acid deficiency, liver disease, reticulocytosis, anticonvulsants, age, smoking, and menopause. Of importance is that the MCV responds slowly to abstinence as well as to relapse to drinking.[9]

High-Density Lipoprotein Cholesterol

High-density lipoprotein (HDL) cholesterol increases as a consequence of excessive alcohol consumption. Other causes for an increase in HDL cholesterol are drugs and vigorous exercise. Furthermore, alcoholic liver injury may decrease the values of HDL cholesterol, a finding that significantly reduces the utility of this marker in actively drinking alcoholics.[13,14]

Ferritin/Transferrin

Serum ferritin may be increased after chronic alcohol consumption. Other conditions in which the serum ferritin is frequently elevated are hemochromatosis, hemosiderosis, liver disease, and inflammatory disorders. As many as 67% of heavy alcohol drinkers with elevated serum GGT levels will also have increased ferritin levels.[15]

Blood Acetate Levels

The elimination of ethanol is enhanced when alcohol is ingested on a regular basis, particularly in chronic alcoholism. This accelerated metabolism of ethanol results in increased levels of the subsequent metabolites of ethanol, acetaldehyde, and acetate. Acetate is formed in the liver from acetaldehyde and is oxidized further to carbon dioxide and water in the peripheral tissues. Acetate is also a normal metabolite in intermediary metabolism, and substantial amounts are formed in the gastrointestinal tract by the microflora. Endogenous acetate levels are low, and during ethanol oxidation, blood acetate rises rapidly and reaches a plateau while ethanol is present. Importantly, blood acetate concentration correlates highly with the rate of ethanol elimination. Consequently, alcoholics have higher blood acetate levels than nonalcoholics. A study found a sensitivity of 65% for blood acetate levels in alcoholics compared with a sensitivity of 64% for serum GGT. The specificity of the blood acetate was 92%.[11,16,17]

Although blood acetate may have clinical utility as a marker for chronic alcohol consumption, it is not specific for chronic alcoholism. Regular users of alcohol may have elevated levels of blood acetate, although they are not alcoholic.[11,17]

Test Combinations

In a large study, the various markers were examined for sensitivity and specificity. Serum GGT was the most sensitive indicator of excessive alcohol consumption—44%. MCV and ASAT were far less sensitive, 16% and 10%, but more specific, 92% and 99%.[18,19]

The sensitivity of the laboratory markers may be improved by using various combinations of GGT, MCV, and ASAT (see Table 5.) The combination HDL cholesterol and GGT has a better discriminitive value in alcoholics than either FFT or HDL cholesterol alone.

A quadratic multiple discriminant function analysis using 24 different laboratory tests classified 100% of medical ward alcoholics as alcoholic and 100% of medical controls as nonalcoholics. However, even with the multiple clinical parameters, the distribution of results between the two patient samples (alcoholic vs. nonalcoholic) overlapped markedly. If the sensitivity was 100%, the best attainable specificity was only about 53%, and if the specificity was 100%, the best sensitivity was 56%.[20,21]

Current Usage of Conventional Testing

The conventional laboratory tests available are useful for alcohol- and drug-related consequences. The laboratory

TABLE 5. Spectrum of Psychiatric Presentations Resulting from Certain Drugs of Abuse

Drug:	Anorexia nervosa	Schizophrenia	Acute psychosis	Major depression	Manic-depression	Personality changes	Organic brain syndrome	Panic, anxiety disorder	Other
Alcohol	+	+	+	+	+	+	+	+	+
PCP	+	+	+	+	+	+	+	+	+
Toluene	+			+		+		+	
Marijuana		+	+	+		+		+	
Amphetamine	+	+	+	+	+	+		+	
Cocaine	+		+	+	+	+		+	
Sedative hypnotics			+	+		+		+	
Heroin				+		+	+	+	
Methadone				+		+	+	+	

tests currently available are not specific for the diagnosis of alcohol and drug addiction. No specific markers exist in conventional laboratory methods or specialized research methods.

The specificity and sensitivity for the conventional laboratory tests are not sufficiently great enough to do mass screening of apparently healthy populations. The present state of knowledge of the biological markers should complement but not replace the measures of alcohol use and the clinical diagnostic criteria for alcoholism and drug addiction.[22,23]

Virtually any psychiatric symptom or syndrome and many medical symptoms and syndromes can be caused by drugs and alcohol. The severity of the psychopathology ranges from mild anxiety and sadness to frank mania and delirium. The symptoms and syndromes caused by drugs and alcohol are indistinguishable from other causes, including the idiopathic origins. The only way to differentiate the etiologies is to identify drugs and alcohol in the history or on drug testing as would be the case with other medical conditions, for example, an infectious process is confirmed frequently by a laboratory method or treated empirically on the basis of the history that is obtained.

The psychiatric syndromes produced by drugs and alcohol are mania, depression, anxiety disorders, personality disorders, schizophrenia, eating disorders, delirium, and dementia (organic mental disorders). The medical symptoms include gastrointestinal, cardiovascular, endocrinological, traumatic, rheumatological, dermatological, and others. These conditions are produced either during the period of drug intoxication or withdrawal or both.[24-31]

Cocaine, for instance, causes mania, personality disturbances, hypertension, cardiac arrhythmias, anorexia, and self-inflicted, excoriating lesions of the skin during intoxication; during withdrawal it produces depression with suicidal thinking, hyperphagia, and hypersomnia.

PCP intoxication produces mania, personality disturbances with violent outbursts, hypertension, cardiac arrhythmias, vivid visual and auditory hallucinations; during
withdrawal it is characterized by depression with suicidal
thoughts. Heroin is associated with endocarditis, arthritis,
and other consequences of intravenous drug use. Inhalation
of organic solvents produces organic brain syndromes such
as delirium and dementia, cardiac arrhythmias, and hepatocellular damage (see Table 4).[32,33-36]

Analytical Testing for the Presence of Alcohol and Drugs

The analytical tests available for drug testing are of two
basic types, chromatographic and competitive-binding/
immunoreactive. The types of chromatographic techniques
are thin layer chromatography (TLC), gas-liquid chromatography (GLC) and high-pressure liquid chromatography
(HPLC), and combined gas chromatography-mass spectrometry (GC/MS). The competitive-binding/immunoreac-
tive techniques are radioimmunoassay (RIA) and enzyme
immunoassay (EIA).[37,24,39]

The sensitivity and specificity of the drug test determines the utility of the test. The tests used for drug testing vary greatly in their sensitivity and specificity.
Unfortunately, some of the laboratory tests used most frequently tend to be low in both sensitivity and specificity.
Moreover, some tests are only qualitative and detect the
presence of the drug without reliable information on the
amount of drug that is present, which becomes important to
differentiate low levels of drugs that persist for prolonged
periods from recent use (Table 6).[37,24,38] The target of drug
testing is either the parent drug or its metabolite. The urine
and blood are assayed, but the urine contains 1,000 times

TABLE 6. Sensitivities of Urine Drug Testing Methodologies (ng/ml)

	TLC	EMIT	GC-MS
Amphetamines	2000	300	25
Barbiturates	2000	300	50
Benzodiazepines	—	1000	50
(Cocaine) BE	2000	75–300	20
Marijuana/THC	20-SP[a]	20–100	20
(Opiates) (Morphine)	2000	300	20
PCP	—	75	20

[a]SP = Special procedure, not detected by routine TLC.

more drug than the blood, so it is preferred as the source to examine. The blood is useful to identify recent use as detection indicates that the drug has not been present long enough to be biotransformed and eliminated from the blood. Moreover, the drug screen is not standard for the number and types of drugs that are assayed, and the types of tests performed for each drug vary from laboratory to laboratory. A clinician must specify the drugs of interest and the types of tests to the laboratory; otherwise only those drugs deemed routine by the laboratory will be done.[37,24,38]

The elimination time of the drug is important to know when a result is likely to be positive for a particular test in relation to the last use. Alcohol is metabolized quickly so that blood and urine are positive for only hours after last use. Metabolites are too common to the body to be reliably measured, that is, acetic acid (Table 7).

The cutoff value is also critical in determining if a drug test is to be reported as positive or negative. The cutoff value is ordinarily selected by the laboratory but can be specified by the physician. Frequently the level is set high to avoid false positives and litigation; however, perfectly valid and reliable results are obtainable if a lower or more sensitive cutoff value is used. A physician can order whatever cutoff value is needed or desired, but it needs to be specified in

Table 7. Cut-off Levels for Detection

Drug	Half-Life (hr)	Emit cutoff (mg/ml)	GC/MS cutoff (ng/ml)	Detectability Range (Days)
1. Amphetamines	10–15	300	100	1–2
2. Barbiturates:				
Short-acting	20–30	300	100	3–5
Long-acting	48–96	—	—	10–14
3. Benzodiazepines:				
Short-acting	20–35	300	—	2–4
Long-acting	50–90	300	100	7–9
4. Cocaine:				
Cocaine	0.8–1.5	—	—	0.2–0.5
Benzodiazepines	—	*300	50	2–4
5. Methaqualone	20–60	300	50	7–14
6. Opiates-codeine-morphine	2–4	300	100	1–2
7. Phencyclidine (PCP)	7–16	75	10	2–8
8. Cannabinoids	10–402	20–100	10	2–8 (acute) 14–42 (chronic)

advance of the testing. A cutoff value of 100 ng/ml will miss many significantly positive samples that a cutoff value of 20 ng/ml would not (see Table 7).[37,24]

The meaning of a positive or negative result is critically important to understand. False negative results are far more common than false positive results. A study done by the CDC (Center for Disease Control) found that 75% of the participating labs reported false negatives on a urine specimen containing 4,000 ng/ml of the cocaine metabolite, far above concentrations that are evident clinically in usual states of use at the time of detection. Another survey by the CDC confirmed the high rate of false negative results by finding 91% of the labs had unacceptable false negative rates for cocaine and benzoylecgonine. Marijuana, PCP, LSD, and other commonly used/abused illicit drugs are not identified at all in most TLC systems. False positive results are quite unusual but can be confirmed with a more specific test such as GC-MS.[39,40]

The confusion arising from the use of drug testing is due to these variables in drug testing in addition to the myriad of clinical variables. Detectability of the drug depends on the type of drug, size of the dose, frequency of use, the route of administration, and the individual variation in drug metabolism. These variables are dependent on the size of the last dose, the sample collection time, and the sensitivity of the analytical method used for drug testing.

TLC has a broad spectrum for drug screening. It is relatively fast and inexpensive but requires an experienced technician to read the TLC plates. TLC is a qualitative test and cannot be quantified so that it yields either a positive or a negative result. The major drawback is its low sensitivity and low specificity. The minimum amount of drug or metabolite necessary to yield a positive result is 1,000–2,000 ng/ml (Table 8).

TLC relies on a reproducible migration pattern by the drug on a thin layer absorbent (e.g., a silica-coated glass

TABLE 8. Sensitivity Levels for Detection

	Sensitivity	
Detection	Ranges (ng/ml)	Cost/sample range ($)
Chromatographic		
TLC	1000–2000	3–10
TLC	10–300	20–40
HPLC	20–300	40–60
GC/MS	5–100	40–100
Immunologic		
EMIT	300–1000	2–6
RIA	2–20	3–10

plate). Characterization of a particular drug is achieved by color reactions produced by spraying the plate with color-complexing reagents. The method was designed to detect very high-dose recent drug use or toxic blood levels from a large variety of drugs. It is a good test for an emergency room, where the drugs taken are unknown and quick determination of *toxic* levels is necessary.[37,24]

Lower levels of drugs that are relevant to producing behavioral changes are not detected with TLC, nor are TLC screens generally admissible as forensic evidence. TLC should be ordered with extreme caution and interpreted with suspicion. Negative results are meaningless by TLC methods, and positive results should be confirmed by a second, more specific method because of TLC's low specificity and sensitivity.[37,24]

GLC is an analytical method that separates molecules by use of a glass or metal tube that is packed with material of a particular polarity. The sample of drug is vaporized at the injection site and carried through the column by a steady flow of gas. The column terminates at a detector that permits recording and quantification. The time to pass through the column is the retention time. A drug has a particular retention time for a given column.

HPLC is similar to GLC. The major difference is the use of liquid rather than a gas to propel the sample through the column in HPLC. Some drug classes are better chromatographed on HPLC (i.e., tricyclic antidepressants and benzodiazepines), whereas other drugs are better detected with GLC, so that they are complementary in a given laboratory. GLC and HPLC are significantly more specific and sensitive than TLC. These methods require extraction, derivatization, column separation, and detection[37,24] (Table 8).

The ultimate laboratory method of detection is by gas chromatography-mass spectrometry (GC-MS). GC-MS analyzes a drug according to its fragmentation pattern. Weaker bonds of the molecules are broken under stress to produce a fragmentation pattern. A perfect match with a fragmentation pattern in a computer library is considered an absolute confirmation of the drug and is referred to as "fingerprinting" of the molecules. The range of sensitivity for the drugs is below 50 ng/ml or 100 to 1,000 times more sensitive and far more specific than the TLC system. Common drugs of abuse and addiction are readily identified in low amounts (i.e., marijuana, cocaine, heroin). The expense of the technique makes GC-MS impractical for screening but vital for confirmation of drug presence and identity (Table 8).[37,24]

RIA and EIA are immunologic methods that employ antibodies against the specific drug and competing drug molecule or enzyme that is labeling with a radioactive tracer. The antibody binding sites are limited in number. The number of radioactively tagged molecules displaced is used to calculate the amount of unlabeled drug in the mixture. The major drawback is the cross-reactivity of drugs and metabolites with the antibodies, which in reality is low. Cross-reactivity can produce a false positive result, but this result can be and should be confirmed by the more specific method, GC-MS. Because the sensitivity is high and the specificity still reasonably high, the EIA and RIA are commonly employed screening techniques. The Enzyme Multiplied Immunoassay Technique (EMIT, trademark of SYVA Co.) is the most widely used methodology for marijuana. The EIA system is very popular because it does not require timely extraction and centrifugation procedures and lends itself to automation.

GC-MS, GLC, HPLC, and some RIA methodologies can be applied to all biologic fluids, including serum. Blood levels are important at times if a clinical state of intoxication is to be correlated with a particular drug in the blood, and blood levels are better indicators of recent use. RIA, EIA, and TLC are not ordinarily designed to detect drug levels in the blood but are used in analyzing urine (see Table 9).[37,24,41]

TABLE 9. Temporal Profile of Drugs Identified by Drug Testing

1. Alcohol—hours
2. Cocaine—hours, days
3. Marijuana—weeks, months
4. Benzodiazepines—weeks, months
5. Opiates—days, weeks
6. Barbiturates—weeks, months
7. PCP—weeks, months

References

1. Salaspuro M: Conventional and coming laboratory markers of alcoholism and heavy drinking. *Alcoholism: Clin and Exp Res* 1986 (Supp); 10(b):5S–12S.
2. Freedland K, Frankel MT, Evenson RC: Biochemical diagnosis of alcoholism in men psychiatric patients. *J of Studies on Alcohol* 1985; 46(2):103–106.
3. Selzer ML: The Michigan Alcoholism Screening Test: The quest for a new diagnostic instrument. *Am J Psychiatry* 1971; 127:89–94.
4. Kristenson H, Trell E, Fex G, Hood B: Serum gammaglutamyl-transferase: Statistical distribution in a middle-aged male population and evaluation of alcohol habits in individuals with elevated levels. *Prev Med* 1980; 9:108–119.
5. Kristenson H, Ohlin H, Hulten-Nosslin MB, Trell E, Hood B: Identification and intervention of heavy drinking in middle-aged men: Results and follow-up of 24-60 months of long term study with randomized controls. *Alcohol Clin Exp Res* 1983; 7:203–209.
6. Morgan MY, Colman JC, Sherlock S: The use of a combination of peripheral markers for diagnosing alcoholism and monitoring for continued abuse. *Journal on Alcohol and Alcoholism* 1981; 16:167–177.
7. Holt S, Skinner HA, Israel Y: Early identification of alcohol abuse. 2. Clinical and laboratory indicators. *Can Med Assoc J* 1981; 124:1279–1294.
8. Rosalk SB, Rau D: Serum gamma-glutamylltranspeptidase activity in alcoholism. *Clin Chim Acta* 1972; 39:41–47.

9. Chalmers DM, Rinsler MG, MacDermott S, Spicer CC, Levi AJ: Biochemical and haematological indicators of excessive alcohol consumption. *Gut* 1981; 22:992–996.
10. Whitefield JB: Alcohol-related biochemical changes in heavy drinkers. *Aust NZ J Med* 1981; 11:132–139.
11. Korri U-M, Nuutinen G, Salaspuro M: Increased blood acetate: A new laboratory marker of alcoholism and heavy drinking. *Alcohol Clin Exp Res* 1985; 9:468–471.
12. Penn R, Worthington DJ: Is serum gamma-glutamyltranspeptidase and alcohol problems. *Lancet* 1981; i:663.
13. Castelli WP, Coyle JT, Gordon T, Hames CG, Hjortland MC, Hulley CB, Kagan A, Zuckel WJ: Alcohol and blood lipids. *Lancet* 1977; ii:153–155.
14. Devenyi P, Robinson GM, Kapur BM, Roncari DAK: High-density lipoprotein cholesterol in male alcoholics with and without severe liver disease. *Am J Med* 1981; 71:589–594.
15. Jacobsson A, Norden A, Qvist J, Wadstein J: Serum ferritin—a new marker for alcoholism? *Acta Soc Med Suec* 1978; 87:3314.
16. Korsten MA, Matsuzki S, Feinman L, Liber CS: High blood adetaldehyde in alcoholics after ethanol administration. *N Eng J Med* 1975; 292:386–389.
17. Nuutinen H, Lindros K, Hekali P, Salaspuro M: Elevated blood acetate as indicator of fast ethanol elimination in chronic alcoholics. *Alcohol* 1985; 2:623–626.
18. Stamm D, Hansert E, Feuerlein W: Excessive consumption of alcohol in men as a biological influence factor in clinical laboratory investigations. *J Clin Chem Biochem* 1984; 22:65–77.
19. Stamm D, Hansert E, Feuerlein W: Detection and exclusion of alcoholism in men on the basis of clinical laboratory findings. *J Clin Chem Clin Biochem* 1984; 22:79–96.
20. Adams KM, Grant I: Failure of nonlinear models of drinking history variables to predict neuropsychological performance in alcoholics. *Am J Psychiatry* 1984; 141:663–667.
21. Eckardt MJ, Feldman DJ: Biochemical correlates of alcohol abuse. In Seixas FA, ed.: *Currents in Alcoholism, Vol. 3, Biological, Biochemical and Clinical Studies.* New York, Grune and Stratton, 1978, 545–554.
22. Jocobson GR: *Alcoholism: Detection, Assessment, and Diagnosis,* New York, Human Sciences Press, Inc., 1976.
23. Ryback RS, Eckardt MJ, Felsher B, Rawlings RR: Biochemical

and hematological correlates of alcoholism and liver disease. *J Am Med Ass* 1978; 248:2261–2265.

24. Verebey K, Gold MS, Mule SJ: Laboratory testing in the diagnosis of marijuana intoxication and withdrawal. *Psychiatric Annals* 1986; 16(4):235–241.

25. Estroff TW, Gold MS: Medication and toxin induced psychiatric disorder. In Extein I, Gold MS, eds.: *Medical Mimics of Psychiatric Disorders.* Washington, DC, American Psychiatric Press, 1984.

26. Estroff TW, Gold MS: Medical and psychiatric complications of cocaine abuse and possible points of pharmacologic intervention. In Stimmel B, ed.: *Advances in Alcohol and Substance Abuse* 1986; 5(1/2):61–76.

27. Estroff TW, Gold MS: Psychiatric misdiagnosis. In Gold MS, Lydiard RB, Carman JS, eds.: *Advances in Psychopharmacology: Predicting and Improving Treatment Response.* Boca Raton, Fl, CRC Press, 1984, pp. 34–66.

28. Weissman MM, Pottenger M, Kleber H, et al: Symptom patterns in primary and secondary depression: A comparison of primary depressives with depressed opiate addicts, alcholics, and schizophrenics. *Arch Gen Psychiatry* 1977; 34:854–862.

29. Thacore VR, Shukla SRP: Cannabis psychosis and paranoid schizophrenia. *Arch Gen Psychiatry* 1976; 33:383–386.

30. Beamish P, Kiloh LG: Psychoses due to amphetamine consumption. *J Ment Sci* 1960; 106:337–343.

31. Extein I, Dackis CA, Gold MS, et al.: Depression in drug addicts and alcoholics. In Extein I, Gold MS, eds.: *Medical Mimics of Psychiatric Disorders.* Washington, DC, American Psychiatric Press, 1986, pp. 133–162.

32. Gold MS, Estroff TW: The comprehensive evaluation of cocaine and opiate abusers. In Hall RCW, Beresford TP, eds.: *Handbook of Psychiatric Diagnostic Procedures.* New York, Spectrum Publications, 1985.

33. Gold MS, Washton AM: *Adverse effects on health and functions of cocaine abuse: Data from 800-Cocaine callers. Trends, patterns and issues in drug abuse,* Vol. 1, Part 2. Rockville, Md. National Institute on Drug Abuse, 1984.

34. Gold MS, Dackis CA, Pottash ALC, et al.: Cocaine update: From bench to bedside. In Stimmel B, ed.: *Advances in Alcohol and Substance Abuse* 1986; 6(2):1–5. New York, Haworth Press.

35. Estroff TW, Gold MS: Chronic medical complications of drug abuse. *Psychiatric Medicine* 1987; 3(3):267–286.
36. Yago KB, Pitts FN, Burgoyne RW et al.: The urban epidemic of phencyclidine (PCP) use: Clinical and laboratory evidence from a public psychiatric hospital emergency service. *J Clin Psychiatry* 1981; 42:193–196.
37. Gold MS, Dackis CA: Role of the laboratory in the evaluation of suspected drug abuse. *J Clin Psychiatry* 1986; 47(1) Suppl:17–23.
38. Gold MS, Pottash ALC, Estroff YW, et al.: Laboratory evaluation in treatment planning. In Karasu TB, ed.: *The Psychiatric Therapies: Part I. The Somatic Therapies.* Washington, DC, APA Commission on Psychiatric Therapies, 1984.
39. *Toxicology, Drug Abuse Survey III: August 19th Proficiency Testing.* Atlanta, GA, Center for Disease Control, 1974.
40. Hansen HJ, Caudill SP, Boone DJ: Crisis in drug testing—Results of CDC blind study. *JAMA* 1985; 25:2382–2387.
41. Gold MS, Pottash AC, Extein I: The psychiatric laboratory. In Bernstein JG, ed.: *Clinical Psychopharmacology.* John Wright PSG., Inc., pp. 29–58, 1984.

9

Diagnosis of Psychiatric Syndromes in Alcoholism and Drug Addiction

A rose is a rose is a rose.

GERTRUDE STEIN

Self-Medication Concept

Alcoholism is considered by some to be secondary to other psychiatric syndromes as an expression of a self-medication of psychiatric symptoms. One origin of the self-medication concept is from early psychoanalytic theory that postulated intrapsychic causes for alcohol use. According to psychoanalytic theory, suppression of unconscious conflict is possible by the tension-reduction effects of alcohol as it is seen as an euphoric and amnestic agent. The alcoholic is seen as having weak ego functioning, that is, unable to integrate and control the powerful forces of the id and the punitive influence of the superego that have developed as a result of unconscious conflicts.

The major difficulties with the psychoanalytic model as an etiological explanation for alcoholism are that the clinical picture of the alcoholic does not correspond to the theory. The disintegrated ego, uncontrolled id, and unbridled superego are a consequence of the addiction to alcohol and not a cause. No studies have confirmed that alcoholics have this or any specific intrapsychic state prior to the onset of alcoholism. On the other hand, many clinical studies and a consensus of clinical impressions have confirmed it as a consequence. Furthermore, once the alcoholism is clearly established, continued alcohol use leads to a worsening, whereas discontinuing it often results in immediate improvement in personality variables.

The biological psychiatry model also relies on the self-medication concept in attributing addictive use of alcohol to underlying affective and psychotic states. A depression is given the antecedent position of causing addictive use of alcohol. Actual experiments performed to study the effect of depression on the drinking behavior of alcoholics and non-alcoholics did not support the hypothesis that depression is a cause of addictive drinking.

Psychiatric symptoms are commonly associated with alcohol and drug use, particularly in chronic addictive use. The relationship between alcohol and drug addiction and idiopathic psychiatric disorders is complex and requires a thorough understanding of both categories of disorders. Not only are the etiology and prognosis of each disorder different, but each requires a unique and sophisticated approach to treatment.[1-4]

Important to bear in mind is that there are no specific symptoms, including alcohol and drug addiction, that are peculiar to only a single psychiatric disorder. Typically, psychiatric symptoms cluster to form psychiatric syndromes in a particular pattern to distinguish one syndrome from another. Furthermore, the relationship between psychiatric symptoms and alcohol and drug addiction provides significant overlap with virtually all of the psychiatric symptoms occurring between them.[5,6] Finally, alcohol and drug addiction is an autonomous and primary disorder with clinical course of its own.

The fundamental criteria of each disorder must be considered before the important aspects of the relationship between the addiction and psychiatric disorders are appreciated. Understanding and utilizing only one approach such as "psychiatric" or "addictive" will yield less success and lead to errors in diagnosis and treatment. The basic definitions of the alcohol and drug addiction and psychiatric disorders must be comprehended before contemplating the diagnosis and treatment.

The acute and chronic use of alcohol and drugs produces signs and symptoms that occur predictably in susceptible individuals, particularly those who have developed an addiction to alcohol and drugs. A review of these signs and symptoms are necessary to appreciate the permutations of syndromes that are induced by alcohol and drugs. Acute use of alcohol and drugs do not ordinarily produce definable psychiatric syndromes beyond intoxication states that persist and require diagnosis and treatment except in exceptional cases of intoxication overdose by the naive user. However, the chronic use of alcohol and drugs is particularly prone to the development of the signs and symptoms that constitute identifiable psychiatric syndromes. Characteristically, these signs and symptoms tend to cluster in aggregates to form a particular pattern as a syndrome for a particular drug or more commonly a combination of drugs and alcohol.[7,10]

Other drugs in addition to alcohol produce the same symptoms that are produced by alcohol. Cocaine, marijuana and phencyclidine (PCP) during intoxication and withdrawal induce intense anxiety and profound depression as well as hallucinations and delusions. The addictive effect with alcohol is expected and does occur regularly. The concurrent use of alcohol and other drugs make it difficult to distinguish between the separate effects of these respective drugs although a clear predominance may emerge with careful inquiry.[11]

Depression

Depression is a common syndrome that is induced by the state of chronic alcohol and drug intoxication. The depression may be mild and intermittent or severe and persistent and is characterized by a lowered mood or decreased spirits and a depressed or constricted affect. Typically, boredom, lack of enthusiasm, energy, and interest in daily living accompany the depressed mood. In more severe cases, frank psychomotor retardation with dulled thought processes, impaired concentration and memory, slowed motor movements, and anhedonia with a lack of motivation for self-care may be manifested.[12–14]

The depression is frequently associated with suicidal ideation, with a high rate of suicide attempts and completion. Twenty-five to 50 of all suicides involve the use of alcohol, often, in alcoholics. One of the single most important risk factors for suicide is alcoholism and drug addiction. A significant proportion, as many as 25% of alcoholics die of suicide as a consequence of their alcoholism. The exact percentage of alcoholics that die of suicide because of associated drug use is unknown but is considered high.[15,16]

Anxiety

Anxiety is also a common disorder that occurs almost inevitably in chronic alcohol and drug consumption. The acute and chronic use of alcohol and many drugs is always accompanied by some discharge of the sympathetic nervous system during the withdrawal state. The sympathetic nervous system, when firing, releases catecholamines that produce the signs and symptoms of anxiety. The spectrum of the anxiety disorders induced by alcohol and drugs is wide and varies from mild anxiety to severe generalized anxiety and phobic states. Virtually all of the states of the "anxiety disorders" can be produced by alcohol and drugs, including generalized anxiety, panic attacks, simple phobias, and agoraphobia. The alcoholic frequently has anxiety and irrational fears that are phobic and range from being afraid to leave the house to a diffuse fear of people, places, and things, for example driving an automobile, appearing in public, socializing in outside drinking situations.[17-24]

These symptoms of anxiety and depression may be particularly troublesome and prompt the alcoholic and drug addict to seek treatment for the anxiety but unfortunately, not the alcoholism and drug addiction. The clinician must be vigilant and attentive to the possibility and likelihood that these symptoms are being produced by alcoholism and drug addiction and their effects. A persistent history with corroborative sources such as the family and employer is often necessary to establish the source of the anxiety as alcoholism and drug addiction.

Hallucinations and Delusions

Classical hallucinations and delusions are less than frequent occurrences in chronic alcoholics and drug addicts although the denial regarding the consequences of alcoholism that is always present in alcoholics and drug addicts is of delusional nature and proportions but not considered a classical delusion. Typically, with alcohol the hallucinations occur as a part of the abstinence syndrome in the form of auditory or visual hallucinations. The *alcoholic hallucinosis,* as it is termed, occurs in a clear sensorium as a part of delirium tremens. The auditory hallucinations are usually of a derogatory nature, condemning and accusatory, and resolve eventually with continued abstinence; however, months may pass before they do. The visual hallucinations are less frequent and are typically, as in delirium tremens, zooscopic in type with animals being visualized, often, insects or rodents or snakes. These also may take months to subside with abstinence from alcohol. [25]

The predominant delusions are paranoid in nature and originate in part from the toxic disturbance of the brain from the alcohol and drugs as do the hallucinations. The delusions take the form of irrational fear that someone or something is out to get the alcoholic and drug addicts. They are a part of the delirium tremens but often occur on their own in a clear sensorium. [25] The cocaine-induced delusional syndrome as characterized by paranoia can persist for days, weeks, or months.

Personality Disorders

The effect on personality by alcohol and drugs is clear and dramatic. Because of the cumulative toxic effects of alcohol and drugs, insight and judgment become impaired and are exercised in improper and self-destructive ways. The typical syndromes of personality disturbances that arise are antisocial, narcissistic, borderline, histrionic, schizoid, dependent, immature, and passive-dependent. The deterioration in personality that occurs as a result of the toxic and addictive process of alcohol and drugs is often devastating. The changes in personality occur insidiously over time and almost imperceptibly at any moment in the progression but become obvious when an interval of time has passed sufficiently for a comparison to be made.

These personality changes are frequently reversible with abstinence and specific treatment for the addiction. For some changes, only a relatively brief time is required for reversibility, whereas other changes in personality may take a prolonged period; months and years may be required after specific treatment of the alcoholisms.[24–28]

Denial

The denial of the alcoholism and drug addiction and its consequences is delusional and can take the form of a fixed, false belief that is irrational and contrary to the evidence. The denial is accompanied by minimization, rationalization, and projection that are utilized to deflect the focus of the alcoholism and drug addiction away from the alcoholic to some other reason or person. Typically, the focus is shifted from the responsibility of the alcoholic to those close to the alcoholic such as a family member, an employer, or "society." When the denial is confronted, it is often resistant to rational evidence of the consequences of the alcoholism and drug addictions. The denial is a mixture of diffuse disruption of the brain from the chemical effect of alcohol and drugs and the intrapsychic, intradynamic defense mechanisms of repression, rationalization, and projection.[29]

Other Causes

The nonspecific nature of the psychiatric symptoms is also seen in other conditions that produce a diffuse disruption of brain function. Primary systemic illnesses occurring throughout the body, affecting the brain secondarily, are common causes of anxiety, depression, hallucinations, and delusions. These symptoms of underlying illnesses are abundant in medical and surgical practices. Primary diseases of the brain such as meningoencephalitis, tumors, and degenerative processes are also common etiologies of anxiety, depressions, hallucinations, and delusions as well.[30]

Idiopathic Psychiatric Syndromes

Idiopathic psychiatric syndromes are typically of unknown origin and consist of signs and symptoms that tend to cluster in a pattern sufficiently common to produce a definable syndrome that serves as a diagnostic category. Anxiety disorders are separated into generalized anxiety, panic attacks, phobic states, and posttraumatic stress disorders. Depression is either termed a major depression as a diagnosis or part of the spectrum of bipolar illness that includes unipolar depression or manic–depressive illness. Schizophrenia is a syndrome of psychotic symptoms such as hallucinations, delusions, and personality deteriortion that may have multiple etiologies as schizophrenia may be a final, common pathway. Personality disorders are many and include antisocial, borderline, histrionic, schizotypal, passive-aggressive, and others. A personality disorder is defined as a collection of personality traits that are maladaptive and develop during early childhood before the age of 15 years old. These traits are constant and enduring and do not vary over time or depend on circumstance for expression. Personality disorders define the individual in a predominant pattern of behavior that is characteristic for that type of personality disorder. Considerable overlap may occur in the personality traits so that multiple personality disorders may occur in the same individual.

Differentiating Induced from Idiopathic Psychiatric Illness

There are guidelines that can be employed to distinguish between the psychiatric syndromes that are caused by

alcohol and drugs and those that exist as idiopathic syndromes by themselves. The first important step is to recognize that, although alcohol and drugs produce psychiatric
syndromes, the reverse that idiopathic psychiatric disorders
cause "addictive" alcohol and drug use is not a clinically relevant approach. Once an addictive pattern has established
itself, the preoccupation with acquiring alcohol, compulsive
use of alcohol, and recurrent relapse to alcohol take prece-
dence over other aspects of the clinical picture and tend to
determine the course of both the addiction and the additional idiopathic psychiatric disorder. The behaviors of addiction are autonomous, having a life of their own, and do
not depend on another psychiatric condition to sustain
them. The addiction supplants the symptoms of the other
disorder to produce a clinical course that will not be altered
significantly by treating only the "underlying," "other," idiopathic psychiatric disorder.

It is clinically useful to separate the two conditions according to their diagnostic criteria, prognosis, and response
to treatment. Although the two are interrelated and affect
the course of the other, keeping in mind the individual characteristics of each is essential to diagnosis and treatment.
The idiopathic psychiatric disorder may or may not predis-
pose to the use of alcohol. The self-medication concept of
"addictive" use of alcohol and drugs is used to explain addictive use, but it fails to account for salient features of
addiction. Both the psychiatrically disordered and the relatively normal individual begin using alcohol and drugs for
similar reasons. The reasons for alcohol use are numerous
and include happiness, sadness, celebration, mourning, vic-
tory, and defeat. The use of alcohol and drugs is often predi-
cated on normal and abnormal states that in themselves are
not specific and distinguishing. At some point, either early
or late in the course of alcohol and drug use, the addictive
process is initiated with the ensuing consequences that are
often psychiatric in nature. The resultant adverse conse-

quences from the addictive process are often worse than the original symptoms that are ascribed as initiating the addictive use. The addiction supersedes the other psychiatric conditions, and the addictive use continues in *spite* of the accruing psychiatric consequences, not because of them.[29–32]

An illustrative example is provided by a study conducted to examine the effect of alcohol on mood. Three groups of subjects were given alcohol to record the response in the mood to the effects of alcohol. The groups of depressed alcoholic, depressed nonalcoholics, and nondepressed nonalcoholics responded differently than expected to the ingestion of a small amount of alcohol. The depressed alcoholic experienced the least benefit with a lowered mood in response to alcohol, whereas the depressed nonalcoholic experienced the greatest improvement in mood followed by the nondepressed nonalcoholic whose mood improvement was between the other two groups.[33]

Furthermore, when the drinking histories of nonalcoholic, manic–depressive individuals are studied, some interesting findings are available. The alcohol consumption of the manic–depressives show no consistent pattern during a depressive episode as it will either decrease, remain the same, or increase. The drinking will increase during a manic phase, most likely consistent with the increased activity of behaviors of many types that are associated with the excesses, indiscretions, and manifestations of poor judgment of the manic state.[33,34]

The conclusions from these studies are that alcoholics continue to drink alcohol *in spite of adverse reactions of mood from alcohol or the alcohol-induced depression and not because of it.* The other important conclusion is that it is erroneous to view addictive alcohol use based on a nonalcoholic experience with alcohol. The nonalcoholic may drink for pleasure or mood elevation but stops short of the adverse consequences because addictive use is not occurring. Ironically, the alcoholic does not appear to "feel good" because drinking makes him or her "feel bad."[33,34]

Studies have characterized the course of depression in alcoholics, particularly, in the active phase of drinking and the acute withdrawal period. These studies have also been performed on chronic users of other drugs such as cocaine, PCP, marijuana, and sedative/hypnotic drugs. The alcohol and drug-induced depression becomes increasingly severe with larger doses and longer duration of use, particularly, heavy, chronic use. The depression often diminishes with decreasing doses and intermittent periods of abstinence and disappears with prolonged abstinence from the alcohol and drugs.[35-38]

In the majority of cases, the depression will remit within days of the cessation of use of alcohol and drugs, although perhaps as many as 10% to 20% of those who are depressed will have a more lasting depression that may take weeks, perhaps months, to subside. Specific treatment of the addiction and additional psychotherapy as needed will usually suffice to treat most cases of lingering depression.[39,40] In a smaller number of cases, 1% to 2%, the depression will persist and require another form of intervention in addition to the treatment of addiction. Antidepressants may be employed in those 1% to 2% of the cases of a persistent depression but are not indicated in the instances of the transient depression, which eventually subsides. Additionally, a large number of alcoholics and drug addicts will have suicidal thinking during the course of the addictive use; some will actually attempt suicide and out of those, some will succeed.

Anxiety is another symptom that is commonly associated with alcohol and drug use and is similar to depression as, the larger the doses and the longer the duration of use, the more frequent and severe the anxiety. The anxiety takes many forms, as previously discussed, and generally will subside with less alcohol and drug use, particularly with some periods of abstinence intermixed. The anxiety tends to remit with time and prolonged abstinence from alcohol and drugs. The acute withdrawal from alcohol and drugs is characterized by intense anxiety, followed by lower intensity over sometimes a protracted course of weeks and months and perhaps years.[18] Persistent, incapacitating anxiety may be treated with low-dose antidepressants with the plan of attempting to discontinue them at some point to determine the continued need.

Laboratory Diagnosis

Laboratory drug testing is a particularly valuable diagnostic tool in evaluating new and old patients and distinguishing between a drug-induced syndrome from an idiopathic psychiatric syndrome (see Chapter 7). At times, the history of drug use is not available or is denied during the interview, and a properly obtained blood and urine screen for drugs is very useful.

The laboratory can aid in making a differential diagnosis and identifying drugs as an active consideration as a cause of psychosis, depression, mania, and personality changes as well as other psychiatric symptoms. Treatment planning and prevention of serious medical consequences often rest on the use of drug screening. Moreover, testing is widely used to monitor progress or relapse in the treatment of alcohol and drug addiction in inpatient and outpatient settings.

The appropriate use of analytic technology in drug testing requires an understanding of available test methodologies. These include drug screening by thin-layer chromatography, comprehensive testing using enzyme immunoassay, and confirmation by gas chromatography–mass spectrometry (GC-MS).

Pharmacological Interventions in Other Diagnoses

Pharmacological intervention is relatively contraindicated in this population as most drugs that are used in the treatment of anxiety such as benzodiazepines are highly addicting in the alcoholic and drug addict. The benzodiazepines and other sedative-hypnotics share pharmacological cross-tolerance and dependence with alcohol. The specific treatment of addiction and other behavioral techniques are most often indicated for the treatment of anxiety in this population.[19,35]

Usually significant anxiety is induced by the alcohol and drugs, although recovery from alcoholism and drug addiction is marked by anxiety and depression from other nonpharmacological causes. The anxiety and depression are due to a number of nonpharmacological reasons derived from the psychological changes that must occur in the recovering alcoholic in order to abstain from alcohol and drugs and the external factors that may have reached crisis proportions because of neglect and poor judgment by the alcoholic and drug addict. These external factors are often difficulties in the areas of major life concerns such as marriage, employment, and legal spheres.

Occasionally, the delusions and hallucinations from alcohol and drugs may persist beyond the period of intoxication and acute detoxification. These symptoms persist uncommonly in alcoholics, although they do occur as in alcoholic hallucinosis. Persisting delusions are more common from heavy, high-dose use of cocaine and PCP and other hallucinogens. These aberrations in thinking are often paranoid in nature and may range from ideas of reference to frank delusions of persecution. A protracted period of weeks to months may be required for these effects from the drugs to subside. If these symptoms are troublesome and of a magnitude that interferes with adequate psychological functioning, short-term use of neuroleptics may be employed to treat the delusions and hallucinations as they occur in the drug-induced states.[41,42]

The use of medications in the alcoholic and drug addict as a rule should be conservative because their basic defect is loss of control over alcohol and drugs. They have similar difficulties in controlling medications they have in controlling alcohol and drugs of addiction. A common attitude among alcoholics and drug addicts is that if one pill works, then two or three must be better. The judgement regarding self-medication in the alcoholic is sometimes as distorted toward medications as it is toward alcohol and drugs of addiction.

Furthermore, most psychotropic medications have adverse sedative and other mood-altering effects on the mentation and emotions of the alcoholic. Antidepressants produce alterations in mood and thinking that may have an adverse pharmacological effect on the alcoholic. Some antihypertensives are sedating and produce aberrations in thinking. There are many other medications that should be used with special consideration and caution in the alcoholic and drug addict. The clinical rule of thumb is that any condition that is not a result of the alcoholism and drug addiction should be treated if required, by weighing the risks and benefits of the use of medications in a population with a relative contraindication for pharmacological effects.

Finally, the signs and symptoms of alcoholism and drug addiction do not respond to pharmacological intervention because there is not specific pharmacological treatment for addiction. The exceptional medication in the treatment of alcoholism may be the use of antabuse as an adjunct to the mainstay treatment of the addiction to reduce the likelihood of impulsive drinking.

The idiopathic psychiatric and medical disorders should be treated as they would be ordinarily with important considerations. The need for medications may be less frequent and in smaller doses when the alcohol and drug use has been eliminated because of diminishing cross-tolerance and dependence. Also the practice of empirical, trial-and-error medicating for atypical symptoms should be avoided in the high-risk population of alcoholics and drug addicts. Importantly, the proper treatment of the additional idiopathic psychiatric disorder is more likely to result in a greater likelihood of success by treating the alcohol and drug addictions. The persistence of a schizophrenic syndrome in an alcoholic will significantly reduce the probability of resisting alcohol use originating from the addictive process. The adequate treatment of a depression will allow the alcoholic to continue to treat the addiction to alcohol. Incapacitating anxiety will also interfere with an acceptable level of functioning in order to abstain from alcohol and drugs. Finally, behavioral programs and intensive psychotherapy may be needed to treat significant personality problems that may be obstructing proper treatment of the alcohol and drug addiction.

References

1. Helzer JE, Przybeck TR: The co-occurrence of alcoholism with other psychiatric disorders in the general population and its impact on treatment. *J Study Alcohol* 1988; 49(3):219–224.
2. Schuckit MA: The history of psychotic symptoms in alcoholics. *J Clin Psychiatry* 1982; 43(2):53–57.
3. Powell BJ, Penick EC, Othmer E, Bingham SF, Rice A: Prevalence of additional psychiatric syndromes among male alcoholics. *J Clin Psychiatry* 1982; 4310:404–407.
4. Wolf AW, Schubert DSP, Patterson MB, Grande TP, Brocco KJ, Pendleton L. Association among major psychiatric diagnoses. *J Consult Clin Psychol* 1988; 56(2):292–294.
5. Schuckit MA: Alcoholism and other psychiatric disorders. *Hosp Community Psychiatry* 1983; 34(11):1022–1027.
6. Schuckit M. Alcoholic patients with secondary depression. *Am J Psychiatry* 1983; 140:6.
7. Miller NS, Gold MS: Suggestions for changes in DSM-III-R criteria for substance use disorders. *Am J Drug Alcohol Abuse* 1989; 15(2):223–230.
8. Jaffe JH: Drug addiction and drug abuse. In Gilman AG, Goodman LS, Rall TW, Murad F, eds.: *The Pharmacological Basis of Therapeutics*, ed. 6. New York, Macmillan Pub. Co., 1985, pp. 532–540.

9. Psychoactive substance use disorders. *Diagnostic and Statistical Manual of Mental Disorders,* 3rd ed. rev. Washington, DC: American Psychiatric Association, 1987, pp. 165–185.

10. Woodruff RA, Guze SB, Clayton PJ, Carr D: Alcoholism and depression. In Goodwin DW, Erickson CK, eds.: *Alcoholism and Affective Disorders.* New York, SP Medical and Scientific Books, 1979, pp. 39–47.

11. Miller NS, Mirin SM: Multiple drug use in alcoholics: Practical and theoretical implications. *Psychiatric Annals* 1989; 19(5):248–255.

12. Schuckit MA: Prevalence of affective disorder in a sample of young men. *Am J Psychiatry* 1982; 139(11):1431–1436.

13. Peace K, Mellsop G: Alcoholism and psychiatric disorder. *Australian NZ J Psychiatry* 1987; 21:94–101.

14. Martin RL, Cloninger CR, Guze SB: Alcohol misuse and depression in women criminals. *J Stud Alcohol* 1985; 46(1):65–71.

15. Martin RL, Cloninger CR, Guze SB, Clayton PJ: Mortality in a follow-up of 500 psychiatric outpatients. I. Total mortality. *Arch Gen Psychiatry* 1985; 42:47–66.

16. Litman RF, Faberow NL, Wold CI, Brown TR: Prediction models of suicidal behaviors. In Beck H, Resnick LP, Lettieri DJ, eds.: *The Prediction of Suicide.* Bowie, MD, Charles Press 1974, p. 141.

17. Small P, Stockwell T, Cantar S, Hodgson R: Alcohol dependence and phobic anxiety states. I. A prevalence study. *Br J Psychiatry* 1984; 144:53–57.

18. Stockwell T, Small P, Hodgson R, Cantar S: Alcohol dependence and phobic anxiety states. II. A retrospective study. *Br J Psychiatry* 1984; 144:58–63.

19. Schuckit MA: Dual diagnosis: Substance abuse and anxiety. The Psychiatric Times 1987; 20–21.

20. Rounsaville BJ, Dolinsky ZS, Babor TF, Meyer RE: Psychopathology as a predictor of treatment outcome in alcoholics. *Arch Gen Psychiatry* 1987; 44:505–513.

21. Stavynski A, Lamontagne Y, Lavallee YJ: Clinical phobias and avoidant personality disorder among alcoholics admitted to an alcoholism rehabilitation setting. *Can J Psychiatry* 1986; 31:714–719.

22. Bibb JL, Chambless DL: Alcohol use and abuse among diagnosed agoraphobics. *Behav Res Ther* 1986; 24(1):49–58.

23. Bowen RC, Cipywnyk CMD, D'Arcy C, Keegan D: Alcoholism, anxiety disorders and agoraphobia. *Alcoholism: Clinical & Experimental Research* 1984; 8(1):48–50.
24. Weiss KJ, Rosenberg DJ: Prevalence of anxiety disorder among alcoholics. *J Clin Psychiatry* 1985; 46:3–5.
25. Adams RP, Victor M: *Principles of Neurology*, 3rd ed. New York, McGraw-Hill, 1985.
26. Mirin SM, Weiss RD: Psychopathology in chronic cocaine abusers. *Am J Drug Alcohol Abuse* 1986; 12(1/2):17–29.
27. Reich J, Chaudry D: Personality of panic disorder of alcoholics. *J Nerv Ment Dis* 1987; 175:224–228.
28. Gawin FH, Kleber HD: Abstinence symptomology and psychiatric diagnosis in cocaine abusers: Clinical observations. *Arch Gen Psychiatry* 1986; 43:107–113.
29. Miller NS: A primer in the treatment process for alcoholism and drug addiction. *Psychiatry Letter* 1987; 5(7):30–37.
30. Petersdorf RG, Adams RD, Braunwald F, eds.: *Harrison's Principles of Internal Medicine*, 10th ed. New York, McGraw-Hill, 1983.
31. Goodwin DW, Guze SB: *Psychiatric Diagnosis*. New York, Oxford University Press, 1980.
32. Milam JR, Ketcham K: *Under the Influence*. Seattle, WA, Madrona Publishers, 1981.
33. Mayfield DG, Alcohol and affect: Experimental studies. In Goodwin DW, Erickson CK, eds.: *Alcoholism and Affective Disorders*. New York, SP Medical and Scientific Books, 1979, Chap. 8, pp. 99–107.
34. Schuckit MA: Alcoholism and affective disorder: Diagnostic confusion. In Goodwin DW, Erickson CK, eds.: *Alcoholism and Affective Disorders*. New York, SP Medical and Scientific Books, 1979, Chap. 1, pp. 9–19.
35. Lader M, Petursson H: Long-term effects of benzodiazepines. *Neuropharmacology* 1983; 22:527–533.
36. Liskow B, Mayfield D, Thiele J: Alcohol and affective disorder: Assessment and treatment. *J Clin Psychiatry* 1982; 43(4):144–147.
37. Post RM, Kotin J, Goodwin FK: The effects of cocaine on depressed patients. *Am J Psychiatry* 1974; 131(5):511–517.
38. Blankfield A: Psychiatric symptoms in alcohol dependence: Diagnostic and treatment implications. *Journal of Substance Abuse Treatment* 1986; 3:275–278.

39. Schuckit MA: The clinical implications of primary diagnostic groups among alcoholics. *Arch Gen Psychiatry* 1985; 42:1043–1049.
40. Miller NS: PCP: A dangerous drug. *Am Fam Physician* 1988; 38(3):215–218.
41. Miller NS, Gold MS, Millman RB: Cocaine. *Am Fam Physician* 1989; 39(2):115–120.

10

Treatment of Alcoholism:
General Considerations

Formula for longevity: Have a chronic disease and take
care of it.

OLIVER WENDELL HOLMES

Does Treatment Work?

Modern and effective treatment for alcoholism and drug addiction does exist and is available to many. The studies that
attempt to determine whether or not alcoholism treatment is
effective vary greatly from researcher to researcher. The
most important variable, however, is the type of treatment
studied.[1,2]

The major difficulties with the studies are that they con-
centrate on a wide variety of treatments administered to an

131

even broader population of alcoholics. The definition of treatment may vary from merely antabuse in a doctor's office with or without Alcoholics Anonymous to a long-term, highly structured, inpatient, 2-year program. Obviously, the treatments are different, and the populations are also disparate as outpatient treatment with antabuse may be aimed at a middle-aged alcoholic with a job and family, whereas the long-term treatment is directed at a young adult, alcoholic heroin addict.[3,4]

Furthermore, as with other medical psychiatric therapies, there is good and bad treatment. Contrary to the notion that treatment is not effective that is widely held within the medical profession, there are essential characteristics that define good treatment. Any physician or other health professional who is seeking treatment for a patient or client will need to be aware of these characteristics. These essential features of effective treatment have been based on actual studies and thousands of patients in clinical experience. As with many medical/psychiatric treatments, clinical trials that include large numbers of patients do not always explain the fundamentals responsible for the success of treatment. At any rate, a key requirement appears to be abstinence from alcohol. Large studies have clearly established that alcoholics cannot be taught to drink with control. Because the fundamental defect in alcoholism is loss of control over alcohol, it is necessary for alcoholics to abstain from alcohol lifelong. In fact, human and animal studies have confirmed that the tolerance to alcohol, and the control of it, diminish with advancing age. The alcoholic who returns to active drinking after a period of many years of abstinence may demonstrate an accelerated decline in the alcoholism, with reduced tolerance and even greater loss of control.

Another fundamental requirement appears to be group therapy, that the alcoholic recover in a group process with other alcoholics. This abiding principle is what is probably the most important aspect of the success of Alcoholics Anonymous, one alcoholic helping another by identifying with each other. The group process is the structure for this to take place in. A facilitator or therapist is needed as a catalyst and director.[5]

Individual therapy is also important, but in the initial stages of therapy for alcoholism it should be supportive, directive, in the "here and now," and designed to motivate the alcoholic to participate in the group process. Insight-oriented and analytical therapies are not indicated in the early treatment of the alcoholic as they may overwhelm him or her who already has severely compromised insight. The alcoholic is filled with remorse and guilt, although this is not always easily seen behind the apparent screen of defiance and belligerence in the state of active alcoholism.[6]

Individual therapy may be indicated for the more severely disturbed and disorganized personality. These particular patients appear to need additional support and guidance because of either a lack of personality strengths or maladaptive behaviors. However, insight and prolonged analytic therapy may be very useful once the alcoholic has achieved some abstinence and commitment to sobriety. The alcoholic may have conflicts that are disturbing and require professional treatment.[6]

The ultimate goal of treatment should be long-term participation and involvement in AA or NA for the alcoholic. The former if the personal preference is alcohol and the latter might be if drugs are the primary experience of the alcoholic. Studies that demonstrate effectiveness of treatment by lengths of abstinence, frequently cite a high correlation between abstinence and attendance at AA. The attendance at AA meeting on a regular basis, at least weekly, is the essential ingredient in maintaining abstinence from alcohol and drugs.[5]

Other factors that promote success but are not absolute

requirements are family support, especially, if the family participates in a recovery program and occupational opportunities and support. Without these factors, the alcoholic may need additional and extended supervised treatment in a so-called "halfway house" or "extended-care" facility. These prolonged stays involve supervised living, with some group and individual therapy, and an emphasis on personal responsibility by having the patient employed in some gainful manner, however modest.[7]

The question of whether outpatient or inpatient treatment is indicated is based on the level of functioning of the individual and the ability to maintain abstinence without an inpatient, structured environment. The alcoholic who is older, more mature, with family support and involvement in treatment, and with less heavy use of drugs and with a job is a more likely candidate for outpatient treatment. Any lack of these variables and a failure of outpatient treatment favor inpatient treatment.[8,9,10]

The outcome data indicate that the alcoholic (and drug addict) who completes a treatment program with these characteristics will achieve and maintain abstinence for 1 year from alcohol and drugs at a rate of 70% if alcohol is the only drug and 60% if both alcohol and drugs are the addictions. The rate of attendance at AA must be at least once a week. Of those who relapse, over half of them will return to abstinence within a few months so that the overall rate of abstinence is high.[11]

According to the General Service Office of Alcoholics Anonymous, if the alcoholic has maintained sobriety for 1 year, the probability is 75% that another year of sobriety will be achieved in AA. If the 2 years of sobriety are achieved, then the probability is 85% that an additional year of sobriety will be achieved. If 5 years of abstinence in AA have been maintained, the probability of another year of sobriety is 98%. AA attendance is assumed in the outcome figures.[12]

Disease Concept

Alcoholism and drug addiction are diseases[13–17] for which treatment is essential and relatively sophisticated.[18] One of the important reasons why Alcoholics Anonymous enjoys the popularity and success that it does today is because of modern and effective treatment for alcoholism. Conversely, treatment for alcoholism has been enhanced by the inclusion of the principles of Alcoholics Anonymous. The two have benefited each other reciprocally. A basic tenet of the treatment approach as in AA is that alcohol and drug addiction are physical, mental, and spiritual diseases. Treatment centers employ physicians, psychologists, counselors, and social workers who treat the diseases of alcoholism and drug addiction. The fundamental treatment focus is on the alcoholic; however, alcoholism (alcohol addiction) is considered a family illness so that the family also is intimately involved in the treatment process. Alcoholism and drug addiction will, and often do, affect each family member as severely and insidiously as they do the alcoholic.[19–22]

Denial and Consequences

Denial in both the alcoholic and the family members is at the basis of the addictions. Without denial, alcohol addiction could not exist in the proportions we know today.[19] There is a significant amount of denial in most alcoholics entering treatment. Contrary to popular belief that the alcoholic has to "want treatment" before it can be effective, almost all alcoholics enter treatment relatively involuntarily. A family member, friend, an employer, or the courts encourage most alcoholics to admit the need for help by confronting the alcoholic with consequence of the alcoholism. Any one or several in combination present the alcoholic with a clear voice: to receive treatment for his or her addictive behavior or if one continues it will mean suffering the consequences of untreated addiction which might be the dissolution of a marriage, loss of a job, or incarceration. This action may be construed as pressure or leverage that "raises the bottom" for the alcoholic before further consequences from alcohol and drug addiction ensue. More accurately, the alcoholic is allowed to face the consequences of his or her addiction. The choice between treatment or the consequences of continued alcohol and drug abuse is for the alcoholic to decide. Unfortunately, the alcoholic frequently does not choose recovery unless the consequences remain in force for refusal of treatment.[17]

The typical alcoholic has a family, job, and a place to live. The alcoholic's functioning is definitely impaired but may still appear adequate by ordinary standards. Total devastation of the alcoholic is not a requirement for admission of a drinking problem and acceptance of treatment for alcoholism. The alcoholic can be persuaded to want help before he or she is rendered permanently, or utterly hopeless, or succumbed to his or her addiction.

Intervention

The technique of intervention in the treatment of alcoholism is a relatively new technique that has been developed in the last 20 years. The clinical dictum that the alcoholic has to want help or reach his or her "bottom" before he or she can recover is only partially true and unfortunately misleading. The alcoholic can be encouraged to accept treatment for his or her alcoholism by intervening or by raising the "bottom" for the alcoholic.

The intervention is often life saving and can initiate a dramatic change in the alcoholics attitude toward accepting treatment. The intervention is an attempt to intervene on the addictive cycle by confronting the alcoholic with the evidence of the consequences of his or her alcoholism. The intervention may be performed by the family, employer, or legal system. Essential to confronting the alcoholic is presenting the alternative for treatment. The consequence for refusal of treatment of the alcoholism may be separation by the spouse, loss of employment, or legal penalty. The ultimate choice lies with the alcoholic.

The members of the intervention team should be willing to express their concerns about the alcoholic with a caring attitude. A condemning and judgmental approach should be discouraged as this is likely to only further alienate the alcoholic and impede any effort to offer him or her treatment. The goal is to allow the alcoholic to face the consequences of his or her illness, and for the enablers to detach from the alcoholic in order for the alcoholic to experience the consequences of the alcoholism.

The purpose of the intervention is an opportunity for the enabler to detach from the alcoholic as much as it is to offer the alcoholic treatment for the alcoholism. The intervention allows the enabler to articulate in a constructive and direct manner concerns that otherwise might be regrets from inaction by the enabler.

The intervention may be organized and led by an experienced clinician or be carried out on a smaller and less formal scale. The intervention may or may not result in an immediate acceptance by the alcoholic of the alcoholism and the necessary treatment. However, it is often a dramatic statement that eventually leads to a desired goal of treatment for the alcoholic.

The intervention may be as simple as the doctor informing the patient of the diagnosis of alcoholism along with the documentation in clinical findings and laboratory confirmation. The physician can also be a potent force in initiating any intervention in concert with family members.

Group Therapy

Much of the treatment process occurs in both large and small groups. These groups are usually directed by a psychiatrist, psychologist, or counselor. Patient interaction is encouraged, and healing occurs when group members reach out to each other. In addiction, identification of one alcoholic with another is a critical step in the alcoholic's ability to accept treatment. The facilitator (a psychiatrist, psychologist, or counselor) guides the patients in supporting and confronting each other. The energy and strength of the treatment process emanate from the group interactions. A profound therapeutic transformation can occur in an individual alcoholic under the influence of the group. The facilitators develop the group's ability to form a cohesive and powerful therapeutic unit. Years of entrenched rationalizations and denial in the alcoholic or drug addict can be dissipated in days or weeks. Honesty and introspection, the bases of recovery, appear. Hope and confidence in the future replaces cynicism. Love replaces hate. The power of the group for healing is endless.

A substantial amount of the treatment process centers around the First Step of AA where the denial of alcoholism and its consequences is gradually confronted. This confrontation of the alcoholic by the group is frequently accomplished by presenting the alcoholic with the evidence of the drinking and drug use that includes the consequences affecting him or her and others. The basic mechanism of denial is a conscious and unconscious self-deception within the alcoholic and the enablers. The enabler is one who protects the alcoholic from the consequences of his or her alcoholism. Another popular term use for enabling is *codependency or coaddiction* because the enabler is dependent on the alcoholic in a reciprocal addictive relationship. The alcoholic and the enabler practice deception to perpetuate the alcoholism. Without this deception, alcoholism could not continue.

The alcoholic and the enabler must deceive themselves and others about drinking and drug use. The antidote to alcoholism and enabling is honesty. An essential and fundamental starting point for recovery from alcoholism and drug addiction in the addict and co-addict is an admission and acceptance of alcoholism and its consequences.

The Twelve Steps

As part of the treatment programs, the first Five Steps of Alcoholics Anonymous may be addressed and completed.

Step One: "We admitted we were powerless over alcohol—that our lives had become unmanageable."[22] The requirement for this step is complete abstinence from alcohol and other drugs to which the alcoholic may be addicted. The alcoholic admits loss of control over alcohol use and accepts the requirement of complete abstinence from alcohol. The alcoholic at some point has lost his or her ability to control the amount of alcohol drunk and the resolve to abstain from alcohol. The word *unmanageable* refers to the effects of alcoholism on the alcoholic and others around him or her. The admission and acceptance of "powerlessness" over alcohol are essential for continued abstinence and change in attitude and mood that occurs as a result of applying the remaining Eleven Steps to the alcoholic's daily life.

The disease concept of alcoholism purports a physical, mental, and spiritual triad,[23,24] referred to as an "allergy" in the original description by psychiatrist Dr. William Silkworth, past medical director of Town's Hospital in New York City. Silkworth bequeathed the disease concept of alcoholism to the cofounders of Alcoholics Anonymous, Bill Wilson and Dr. Robert Smith, who incorporated it into the program of recovery of AA.[22]

Well-known toxic consequences of alcohol on the brain and body have been described in detail in a variety of medical sources.[25,26] These physical and neuropsychological consequences of alcohol use include widespread involvement of many organ systems in the body.[27–32] Cognitive, mood, and memory disturbances emanate from direct toxic perturbations of the brain cells in a diffuse distribution in both higher cerebral and lower limbic centers.[33] A multitude of medical sequelae ensue from disruption of function, and at times pathological injury, in the gastrointestinal, cardiovascular, pulmonary, endocrine, and integumentary systems as well as others.[34]

The mental consequences are dramatically illustrated in the psychological state of the alcoholic that contains many paradoxical characterizations. The outer phenomenology provides a protrait of a defiant, overconfident, exuberant, and independent personality behind which is a victim who feels inferior, depressed, dependent, hopeless, helpless, and worthless. The disease of alcoholism (and drug addiction) has rendered the individual powerless over alcohol and self. An added mental agony is that the alcoholic (addict) is at least partially aware of the hopelessness of this predicament but is unable by resolve and will to deter his or her apparent self-inflicted demise.[17,19]

The spiritual consequences are devastating. Usually, the alcoholic has been acting and thinking contrary to his moral standard or values, that is, sense of right and wrong, which has produced a significant sense of guilt and isolation from himself/herself and others. The price of denying his or her conscience its proper and sufficient expression is enormous and uncompromising. The existential state of the alcoholic is to not believe in any power that is greater than himself/herself to maintain the illusion of self-reliance and the pattern of addiction that is loss of self-control. The chaos produced by the alcoholic's exercising his or her self-will in the face of an overpowering addiction is evident in all aspects of his or her attitudes, moods, and perceptions. The complexity of the addictive state is greater than the simple inebriation from alcohol and drugs; the sense of "being" is corrupted. The sense of well-being is replaced by a profound loss of meaning. Self-centered purpose and direction masquerade as a contemporary justification of Machiavellian thinking and action.

A profound lowering of mood and a change in self-attitude of worthlessness, hopelessness, helplessness, and self-blame constitute a syndrome of depression, sometimes very severe. Disturbances in vegetative functions such as altered sleep and eating patterns may occur. A blunted affect and psychomotor retardation may accompany the depressive state induced by alcoholism and drug addiction. The specific treatment of the alcohol and drug addiction with abstinence and the addict's application of the steps will often relieve and resolve the severe depressive syndrome. Action taken in these steps will often result in an elevation of mood and an establishment of an improved self-attitude. Spontaneous and expressive affect and behaviors replace the earlier dour and downtrodden appearance. Abstinence and the Twelve Step Program frequently are not only necessary but sufficient for the reversal of "endogenous" or "biological depressions." The Dexamethasone Suppression Test and Thyroid Releasing Hormone Test are frequently abnormal in active alcoholics and drug addicts and normal during abstinence; this suggests an alcohol and drug-induced biological substrate for the major depression seen in this population.[19]

A common conclusion and an almost natural sequelae to the cumulative effects of the physical, mental, and spiritual deterioration and degradation induced by alcohol and drugs is suicidal thought and sometimes actions. Next to advancing age, alcoholism and drug addiction are the most serious risk factors for suicide, at least equal and probably above idiopathic depression that occupies a lower position among risk factors.[35,36]

The adverse consequences are evident in the disruption of family harmony and cohesiveness; impaired performance

at work, an array of legal entanglements and social infringe-
ments; and a wide variety of personal indiscretions and vi-
olations. These add to the already substantial guilt and
isolation of the alcoholic.

The alcoholic now experiences a severe impairment in
the perception of his or her "reality" and in the ability to discern and judge accurately. If honesty or self-insight uncovers
this state of powerlessness and irrationality, then the need
for a power greater than the alcohol and drugs is required to
relieve the insanity of continued addictive use.

Step Two: "Came to believe that a power greater than
ourselves could restore us to sanity."[22] The alcoholic willpower, wits, and character are unable to keep from drinking. The alcoholic, in reality, drinks addictively against his
or her will. Even knowing the consequences of another bout
of drinking and the loss of control if even one drink is taken,
the alcoholic frequently will pick up the first drink that sets
into motion an unyielding, compulsive consumption of alcohol. The alcoholic has lost the willpower to refuse a drink or
a drug. The dilemma of the alcoholic is a lack of power of
choice to avoid drinking and drug use that is the basis of an
addiction. Furthermore, the misconception that the alcoholic
enjoys drinking at the point of addictive use perpetuates the
moral condemnation of the alcoholic. The euphoria or enjoy-
ment has usually long waned from the drinking experience
of the alcoholic. The mystery is that the alcoholic continues
to drink without pleasure, despite the anhedonia produced
by addictive drinking.

An addiction has three components: a preoccupation
with alcohol (and other drugs), compulsive use, and relapse
to alcohol (and drugs). In order for the alcoholic to suc-
cessfully resist the addiction, outside help must be accepted. The insanity is that the alcoholic drinks even though
to drink may mean significant adverse consequences and
perhaps death, slow or fast; however, the alcoholic will often
drink simply because of the addiction. Paradoxically, the

power utilized by the alcoholic can only be other than or outside the alcoholic. The power, while under treatment, is often the physician or counselor, or the group of alcoholics in the treatment program at the time. The power begins with the acceptance of the alcoholism and is frequently accompanied by the confidence and hope that there is a solution to alcoholism and drug addiction that is attainable for the alcoholic. A detailed explanation of the solution is not necessary for acceptance of the therapy. Before further progress is made, a belief in that power outside the alcohol is needed. The belief begins by a decision to use the power as "understood by the alcoholic."

Step Three: "Made a decision to turn our will and our lives over to the care of God *as we understood Him.*" No attendance in a church or adherence to theological dogma is required to accomplish this step; only a decision. The important factor in initiating this step is for the alcoholic to make a decision to turn his or her "will and life" over to the care of God. This step is not religious in nature. The alcoholic volunteers some confidence and faith that accepting therapy for the alcoholism will work. The requirement is to "make a decision" to accept help from a power greater than himself or herself. An important and critical issue of this step is control. Repeatedly the alcoholic has failed at efforts to control his or her drinking patterns and alcoholism and has made persistent, although unsuccessful, attempts to control time, quantity, and places of alcohol and drug consumption. More importantly, the emotional control and "instincts" that have gone awry have produced a state of fury and confusion in the alcoholic. The need for sex, food, love, and security has been often exaggerated, distorted, and misdirected by the alcohol and drugs, sometimes into forms of other illnesses such as sexual and eating disorders. The basis of these distortions in sex, food, and emotions is multigenic, derived from disturbances in the limbic system by the toxic effects of alcohol and drugs. The limbic system contains the neuro-substrate for emotions (such as anger, placidity, fear), sexual drive and expression, hunger, and memory.[33,37] The drive states and emotions may have been entrained by, and associated with, alcohol and drugs. A reduction in the drive state may be satisfied by the reinforcement produced by alcohol and drugs.[34]

A caricature develops of a self-centered, immature, self-seeking, self-willed, narcissistic, passive-dependent, hysterical, antisocial, and paranoid personality. A defiance of the superego and its punitive exhortations is costly in the degree of guilt that is inflicted on the victim. The addictive process that forces the individual to defy important moral values and ethical directives provokes the superego. The id is allowed a freer expression of primitive impulses by the disinhibiting effects of alcohol and drugs. The cumulative effect is destructive and overwhelming to the ego that is attempting to "control" all the diverse impulses and conflicts.

The alcoholic must paradoxically relinquish these attempts at control to regain mastery over self, emotions, and instincts. The belief that a power both spiritual and human will return the control to the alcoholic is an essential step in recovery. A self-trust begins with a trust in others, both visible and invisible. The key phrase in this step is God "as we understand Him," where the alcoholic chooses to apply his or her will to a source of strength and help other than the addictive mode directed by the drives in the limbic system that has been occupying his or her attitude, mood, and perceptions.

Step Four: "Made a searching and fearless moral inventory of ourselves."[22] This step requires recounting and detailing the consequences of the alcoholism and drug addiction admitted in the First Step. The alcoholic takes an inventory of the way in which alcohol has adversely affected him or her and others. The expression of conscious and unconscious material to the self is of paramount importance for the alcoholic to achieve a psychodynamic equilibrium. The inventory pertains to conscious and unconscious conflicts that represent the obstacles that may or may not include moral judgments, within the alcoholic to future recovery. These obstacles frequently include defects in emotions (mood) and attitudes such as resentments, anger and fears, immaturity, and sources of guilt. Some mastery over emotions, change in attitudes, and resolution of guilt must occur for the alcoholic to achieve and maintain recovery, enjoy satisfactory sobriety, and to avoid the syndrome of "depression" that is the total expression of these derangements in emotions, attitudes, and guilt. A self-mastering over the limbic system by higher cortical function is promoted by the use of the intellectual and spiritual exercise of self-inventory. Cerebral centers must ultimately dominate over brain stem function. Neocortical inhibition of the phylogenetically primitive limbic impulses must occur for the addiction to be arrested.

Step Five: "Admitted to God, to ourselves, and to another human being the exact nature of our wrongs."[22] This is a step of confession or in psychodynamic terms, a release of conscious and unconscious conflict to achieve an intrapsychic equilibrium between ego, id, and superego. The alcoholic confides in and confesses to someone else the obstacles in the form of distorted attitudes and deranged morals uncovered in Step Four. This is a necessary step for the alcoholic to achieve full awareness regarding his or her intrapsychic state and effect of the consequences of the alcoholism. Confidentiality is a critical requirement for this step. A skilled and compassionate listener, knowledgeable to the purpose of the alcoholic, is essential. The other person frequently is a sponsor in AA or a clergyman, although it can be a psychiatrist or counselor. The confession is therapeutic by itself, relieving depressive moods and distorted attitudes and frequently leads to a solid foundation for recovery if done with a measure of honesty and sincerity.

Alcoholism as a Family Illness

The family undergoes a similar clinical evaluation, self-scrutiny, and treatment. The family members must examine their state of denial and how the disease of alcoholism and drug addiction has affected them over the years. Those non-alcoholics affected by alcoholism are said to be as "ill" as the alcoholic. The recognition of their illness is often difficult because the identification of the alcoholic as the primary problem tends to distract attention from the nonalcoholic and to disguise the severe personality disturbances that can occur in those affected by the alcoholic. Often resentments that are directed toward the alcoholic are key offenders present within the family.

It is critically important for the entire family to be included in the treatment process at the same time as the alcoholic. Not doing so can delay not only the alcoholic's progress but can also delay the treatment of the family. Alcoholics who are more likely to recover are those who have the support and involvement of their family and significant others. The alcoholic who is alone without family, social, and community support is statistically less apt to recover. The more the family knows and the healthier it becomes through treatment, the better able the alcoholic and the family are to recover together.[19,22]

Treatment of Coaddiction

A fair statement is that without an enabling society and family, alcoholism and drug addiction could not exist, at least, in the proportions they do today. The attitudes on the part of others are critical in the initiation, evolution, and maintenance of alcoholism. As outlined in the chapter on prevention, the exposure to alcohol is determined by society and the family. The ground rules for use and the expectations of the practices surrounding alcohol and drug use are set by all of us. Of course, there are legal stipulations that govern the use and overuse of alcohol and drugs.

These laws merely reflect the mood and will of society, and in themselves do not contain intrinsic meaning beyond what society will allow. The enforcement of these laws also depends on the expectations of society and the census of its members, manifested by what it will tolerate within and outside the law.

The enabling extends further beyond the sociological and legal limits of alcohol and drug use and affects the everyday practices of the individual. Enabling is defined as allowing the use of alcohol and drugs. The allowing of the use of alcohol and drugs may or may not be responsible or be done in a responsible manner. In fact, the enabling may extend into encouraging the use and overuse of alcohol and drugs. The enabling may become a part of a complex, overall relationship between the user and the enabler. This relationship becomes detrimental to both the alcoholic and the enabler. The enabler may take on typical characteristics that form a syndrome, entitled *codependence* or *coaddiction.*

The enabling system is particularly potent during the years when drinking and drug use is introduced in adolescence. The peer pressure to not only try but to use alcohol and drugs on a regular basis is large and powerful. The threat of loss of acceptance and expulsion from one's own group is a force that is compelling to the individual to use alcohol and drugs. Those who resist society's demand to use alcohol and drugs run the risk of being stereotyped in ways that do not accurately reflect them and may actually restrict them in important ways in their efforts to succeed in society at that time.

Because the age of risk for alcoholism and the peak period for the age of onset of alcoholism is in adolescence and early adulthood, the attitudes and practices regarding alcohol and drug use are critical during these important formative years. At present, our society has definite improvement to make in order to reduce the enabling system for the adolescent and young adult. Sporting events, either for participation or spectating, are saturated with exhortations to use and to use alcohol often. Because alcohol is a drug, the message may be interpreted to include other drugs. It has only been recently that cigarette smoking has been determined to be a drug addiction. Marijuana is not even considered to be a drug by many. With these prevailing attitudes, the limits and enforcement of laws are obscure and difficult.

Another unfortunate attitude toward alcohol and drug use and addiction is that it is only the responsibility of the individual and that others do not have any responsibility beyond the individual. The errors in this line of reasoning are many. As discussed, the limits imposed by society for use and practices regarding alcohol are each individual's responsibility as being a part of that society. Furthermore, the ways in which alcoholism is diagnosed and treated are within the bounds of society, particularly the medical profession.

The basic reason why alcoholism is left to the individual to take care of is that it is not considered an illness or disease. Society shares in the responsibility of the diagnosis and treatment of illnesses, but it assigns those conditions that are considered immoral or illegal to the individual. Because alcoholism is a physical, mental, and spiritual illness, it needs to be diagnosed and treated as another illness. Alcoholism and drug addiction are the kinds of illnesses that cannot be left to the individual. The individual without help cannot recover from alcoholism and drug addiction just as someone with pneumonia cannot recover without proper treatment.

The family and employer are two institutions that are especially susceptible to the development of the coaddiction or codependence syndrome. These conditions are the parallels to alcoholism and drug addiction in those who are in a relationship with the alcoholic and drug addict. Codepen-

dents or coaddicts develop a similar denial and other intrapsychic dynamic that is present in the alcoholic and drug
addict.

The denial is generally of the alcoholism and drug addiction as well as the consequences. If a problem with drinking is acknowledged to exist, the practice is to attribute the
alcoholism to another condition or cause. A common practice is to assign the consequences as the antecedent, such
that the marital discord and depression are the cause of the
drinking. The proper sequence is usually that the alcohol
consumption is causing or at least contributing and preventing a resolution to the marital problems and most often
causing the depression.

The denial is both conscious and unconscious and is directed at maintaining an equilibrium within the enabler. Unfortunately, the denial is counterproductive for both the
alcoholic and the enabler as the alcoholism and drug addiction are allowed to continue as long as the true nature and
importance of the alcoholism is not recognized and treated.

Other defense mechanisms that are active and counterproductive are minimization, rationalization, and projection. Minimization is lessening or deemphasizing the
severity and consequences of the alcoholism in order to
seemingly protect the alcoholic and drug addict. However,
the more the consequences are minimized, the less apt an
accurate assessment and proper treatment will be instituted.
The rationalization is part of the tendency to make excuses
for the alcoholic and to cover up for consequences of alcoholism. The most effective means of treatment of alcoholism is
to allow the alcoholic to face and accept the consequences of
the alcoholism fully and squarely, along with the treatment.
If the alcoholic refuses treatment, then the full force of the
consequences of alcoholism should be allowed to take effect.
If treatment is accepted, then some measure of allowance
that the consequences originated from an illness can be included in the deliberation of the final measure of the conse-

quences. A frequent example is an alcoholic who faces the prospect of losing a job or marriage or a legal consequence as a result of alcoholism. If the alcoholic accepts treatment and the offer for help, then the employment may be continued as long as the alcoholism remains in remission. Likewise, the spouse of the alcoholic may want to continue a marriage as long as the alcoholic is able to treat his or her alcoholism. Finally, a court sentencing may include in it consideration of retribution that the alcoholic expresses regret and intends to make amends by accepting treatment of the alcoholism and drug addiction.

Projection is a defense mechanism in which the feelings and thoughts of an individual are displaced or projected onto another individual. For instance, in the case of the alcoholic, projection allows for the inability to accept responsibility for the alcoholism and the consequences of the alcoholism and the assignment of blame outside the alcoholic and away from the alcoholism. The enabler uses the same projection to escape the responsibility for a part in the support and propagation of the alcoholism. The enabler blames the alcoholic for his or her shortcomings and projects resentment onto the alcoholic.

Perhaps the critical observation that can be made regarding the enabler–alcoholic relationship is that the enabler focuses on the alcoholic and not on him- or herself. The enabler becomes addicted to the alcoholic in a way that satisfies the criteria for addiction; hence, the term *coaddiction*. The enabler becomes preoccupied with the alcoholic, and in fact the alcoholic becomes an obsession to the enabler. The enablers are vulnerable to persistent intrusions into their moods and thoughts, in such a way that the alcoholic controls the moods and thoughts of the enabler, even when this influence is not consciously wanted.

The enabler also continues to compulsively pursue and protect the alcoholic in spite of numerous adverse consequences from the alcoholism. The enabler is unable to refrain from performing specific acts that allow the alcoholic to continue to use alcohol and drugs. The enabler may even feel uneasy when the alcoholic abstains or shows signs of wanting to recover. The enabler, because of the addiction to the alcoholic, is unable to stop enabling the alcoholic in the same way the alcoholic is unable to stop without help.

Finally, the enabler may for periods of time be able to not allow the alcoholic to drink or use drugs. However, as with any addiction, the enabler eventually relapses into some behavioral pattern that allows the alcoholic to avoid the consequences of the alcoholism. At that point, the alcoholic can continue to drink because of the assistance from the enabler.

The enabler often needs treatment for the enabling in the same way that the alcoholic needs treatment for the alcoholism. The enabler's denial and minimization need to be confronted as in the case of the alcoholic. The enabler needs to detach from the alcoholic in order to discontinue the addictive cycle.

There are specific programs available that treat the coaddiction component of the overall disease of alcoholism. Many treatment programs for alcoholism include a family program directed specifically at the coaddiction as a family disease. There are also specific programs intended for the enabler in which therapy is for the coaddict only. Al-Anon is one such program that is available to anyone who needs treatment for enabling and coaddiction.

Aftercare

Alcoholism is a lifelong disease, and treatment cannot end at the unit door. The cornerstone of successful treatment is participation by the patient and family in an aftercare program. As President Reagan said to Gorbachev, "trust but verify," so too does aftercare mean meetings and urine testing—and then more meetings and urine testing.

The vast majority of these programs are affiliated with Alcoholics Anonymous, and the 12-step recovery program pioneered by that organization has since been used in a wide variety of addiction treatments. A parallel program for families, Al-Anon, also embraces AA's 12-step program but focuses on the "codependent" family member.

Follow-up and continued treatment after discharge from an inpatient program for alcoholism and drug addiction can contain a variety of ingredients. It may be only an entrance into Alcoholics Anonymous in the community as a continuation by the alcoholic who began attending AA meetings while in treatment. The family members and significant others who are not alcoholic are encouraged to attend Al-Anon on a regular basis. Some alcoholics need placement in residential treatment facilities that are called "halfway houses." This is a misnomer because these facilities are actually extended treatment care facilities where the alcoholic continues to receive group therapy and individual counseling, has employment, and attends meetings of Alcoholics Anonymous.

Day or partial hospital treatment programs are currently available in some centers. These programs provide the full range of group and individual therapies that are available to the inpatients and outpatients. The patients may have completed inpatient programs and have progressed to a stable state not requiring the therapeutic structure of a full-time stay in the hospital. Patients may also attend partial or day hospital programs *de novo* without a prior inpatient program if their clinical state and social supports are sufficiently stable to promote abstinence from alcohol and regular attendance in the program.

For many alcoholics, aftercare treatment on a follow-up basis after discharge from a hospital program is important and often involves the family. The treatment program may include discussions, education, and group therapies that address current problems shared by the alcoholics and their families. These are more than support groups. They are actual therapy groups that meet on a regular basis between one to five times a week with a duration of 1 or more hours a day or evening. The total duration of treatment may be weeks, months, or years.

In addition, alcoholics have other psychiatric problems more frequently than other populations that include eating, sexual, mood, and personality disorders that can also be addressed in the hospital programs and in the follow-up treatment plans. Special types of treatments and therapies from psychiatrists and psychologists are available for these recovering alcoholics and drug addicts. There are also support groups in the community for bulimics, anorexics, and individuals with particular sexual problems.

Alcoholics Anonymous

Alcoholics Anonymous (AA) is a fellowship of men and women whose primary purpose is to remain abstinent from alcohol and to assist other alcoholics to achieve sobriety. Alcoholics Anonymous is a worldwide organization with a membership estimated in the millions. Meetings are held on a daily basis throughout the day, evening, and night in virtually every city in the United States. There are thousands of meetings of Alcoholics Anonymous a week in the five boroughs of New York City. A central clearinghouse for Alcoholics Anonymous is located in each city for the place and times of local meetings. This office is listed in the white or yellow pages of the telephone book under AA or Alcoholics Anonymous.[38]

The only requirement for membership in Alcoholics Anonymous is the desire to stop drinking alcohol. Many AA members have additional drug problems as well, such as marijuana, cocaine, barbiturates, or other drug use. Membership in Alcoholics Anonymous is strictly confidential and voluntary. No attendance is taken, though some groups may have an optional roster list with names, addresses, and phone numbers for reference by members. Although there is no regularly scheduled contact for members between meetings, members irregularly initiate contact with each other for friendship, fellowship, or concern. The meetings generally have a composition that includes both sexes and a wide range of ages, occupations, nationalities, and socioeconomic backgrounds. The strongest meetings have the largest and most varied mixture. A typical meeting currently may include business people, housewives, professionals, students, the retired, and unemployed, with any age represented (the average age of entry into AA is 30 years old, with about 60% men and 40% women).[12]

The largest age group represented is 31–50 with 52%, followed by 51 and over with 28%, 30 and under with 20%, and 21 and under with 3% (but increasing). At a typical AA meeting, the duration of sobriety (i.e., continuous abstinence from alcohol and other drugs) is 35% to 40% sober less than 1 year, 35% to 40% sober 1 to 5 years, and 20% to 30% sober over 5 years.[40]

The routes of entry or referral for the AA member are by another AA member, 37%; self, 27%; through treatment or rehabilitation centers and counseling, 31%; a family member, 20%; by a physician, 7%; through correctional institutions, 4%.[39]

The "typical AA member" in 1984 as surveyed by the AA world services had the following characteristics: sobriety to date—45 months; percentage of women, 30%; average meetings a week—4; having prior counseling—60%; addicted to another drug—31%. Since 1984 the major trends have been toward longer sobriety, greater proportion of women, and greater numbers who are addicted to another drug.[39]

The meetings are held in a variety of facilities—schools, churches, hospitals, and members' homes. The meetings are noted in published schedules and registered with Intergroup or the central office. Many are listed with the General Service Office in New York City.

Service Structure. The General Service Office (GSO) is the organizational hub of the complex General Service Structure, which coordinates the districts, areas, and regions that represent individual AA groups worldwide.[12] At the top of this managerial framework is a Board of Trustees overseeing all operations.

The AA groups are divided into districts, areas, and regions for purposes of consolidating the leadership and decision-making functions. Each level of organization has officers and committees. The basic unit of this structure is the general service representative from each AA group. The AA groups are merged into districts, usually according to population and geography; and these districts into larger assemblies. These area assemblies are represented by elected delegates, similar to congressional representatives from "congressional districts."

Delegates attend the General Service Conference held in New York City annually; a meeting that is representative of the AA "group conscience as a whole." The General Service Conference makes recommendations to the Board of Trustees. Areas are joined into larger regions from which trustees are chosen. The trustees meet regularly as a board that is responsible for determining policies. Most of the leadership including delegates and trustees are elected by a parliamentary process. The General Service Office in New York City employs a number of full-time professionals. Many but not all of the Board of Trustees and the staff are recovering alcoholics. GSO as well as the Board of Trustees have always employed a number of nonalcoholics.[12]

Group Structure. The AA group is autonomous in all its affairs. The leadership, including the General Service Structure, are considered "trusted servants." The AA group functions according to the 12 traditions that are suggestions rather than mandates for procedures and operations. These traditions insure the integrity of the AA groups and by doing so, the AA movement and organization as a whole. The group interprets the traditions according to the "group conscience" that allows for individual application of the traditions.

Individual Structure. The AA member maintains abstinence from alcohol and other drugs and recovers physically, mentally, and spiritually according to the Twelve Steps. These steps are spiritual and behavioral in nature and are designed to induce a fundamental change in attitude, personality, and mood in the recovered alcoholic. The First Step requires abstinence from alcohol and other drugs as a beginning. The remaining steps are principles for achieving and maintaining an adequate attitude and mood for satisfactory interpersonal relationships.

These principles embodied within the Twelve Steps are intended to denote that action must be taken to recover from alcoholism. The alcoholic "acts" his or her way into "proper attitudes and moods" rather than contemplates a change to promote new behaviors. The steps are prescriptions to "perform" a transformation in personality. Basic conflicts, rooted in the past and present, can and must be resolved before a sufficient emotional state is reached to aid the alcoholic in resisting the preoccupation with, compulsive use of, and eventual relapse to alcohol and/or drugs.

Relationship between AA and Treatment

The principles and philosophy of the abstinence-based Twelve Steps Program of Alcoholics Anonymous can be incorporated into the treatment process for alcohol and drug addiction. Current inpatient and outpatient psychiatric treatment may utilize the first five steps as an approach to alcohol and drug addiction. Furthermore, the program of Alcoholics Anonymous is recommended as a mainstay of continued treatment in the long-term follow-up. However, neither AA nor the treatment or rehabilitative centers have any affiliation with each other as suggested in the Sixth Tradition.

References

1. Emrick DC: Evaluation of alcoholism therapy methods. In Pattison EM, Kaufman E, eds.: *Encyclopedic Handbook of Alcoholism.* New York, Gardner Press, 1982.
2. Jones KR, Vischi TR: Impact of alcohol, drug abuse and mental health treatment on medical care utilization: A review of the research literature. *Med. Care* 1979; 17 (suppl.):1.
3. Polich JM, Armor DJ, Braiker HB: *The Course of Alcoholism: Four Years After Treatment.* New York, Wiley, 1981.
4. Plotnick DE, Adams IM, Hunter HR, et al.: *Alcoholic Treatment Programs Within Prepaid Group Practice HMO's: A Final Report.* Contract No. ADM 281-80-004, prepared by the Group Health Association of America for National Institute on Alcohol Abuse and Alcoholism, Alcohol, Drug Abuse, and Mental Health Administration, May, 1982.
5. Miller NS: A primer for the treatment of alcoholism and drug addiction. *Psychiatry Letter* (Fair Oaks Hospital) July 1987.
6. Hill MJ, Blane HT: Evaluation of psychotherapy with alcoholics. *Q J Stud Alcohol* 1967; 28:76.
7. Voegtlin W, Lemere F: The treatment of alcohol addiction: A review of the literature. *Q J Stud Alcohol* 1942; 2:717.
8. Brandsma J, Maultsby M, Welsh R: *Outpatient Treatment of Alcoholism: A Review and Comparative Study.* Baltimore, University Park Press, 1980.
9. Holder DH, Hallan JB: *A Study of Health Insurance Coverage For Alcoholism For California State Employees.* Unpublished report to the National Institute on Alcohol Abuse and Alcoholism, Alcohol, Drug Abuse, and Mental Health Administration, December, 1976.
10. Wanberg KW, Horn JL, Fairchild D: Hospital versus community treatment of alcoholism problems. *Int J Ment Health* 1974; 3:160.

11. Laundergan JC: *Easy Does It, Alcoholism Treatment Outcomes.* Hazelden, MN, Hazelden Foundation, 1982.
12. General Service Office Alcoholics Anonymous, P.O. Box 459, Grand Central Station, NY, NY.
13. Edwards G, Arif A, Hodgson R: Nomenclature and classification of drug and alcohol related problems. *Bull WHO* 1981; 59:225–242.
14. Jellinek EM: The disease concept of alcoholism. New Brunswick, NJ, Hillhouse Press, pp. 139–148, 1960.
15. Vaillant GE: *The Natural History of Alcoholism,* Cambridge, Harvard University Press, 1983.
16. Milam JR, Ketcham K: *Under the Influence.* Seattle, WA, Madrona Publishers, 1981.
17. Gold MS, Verebey K: The pharmacology of cocaine. *Psychiatric Annals* 1984; 14(10):714–723.
18. Dackis CA, Gold MS, Estroff TW: Inpatient treatment of addiction. *In Treatment* of Psychiatric Disorders: *A Taskforce Report of the American Psychiatric Association,* Vol. 2, 1989:1359–1379.
19. Milam J: *The Emergent Concept of Alcoholism.* Kirkland, WA, Alcoholism Center Associates, Inc., Press, 1978.
20. Mendelson JH, Mello NK: *The Diagnosis and Treatment of Alcoholism.* Ed. 2. McGraw-Hill, New York, 1985.
21 Goodwin DW: Familial alcoholism: A review. *J Clin Psychiatry* 1984; 45(12):14–17.
22. *Alcoholics Anonymous,* 3rd ed. New York, Alcoholics Anonymous World Services, Inc., 1976.
23. Jellinek EM, Jolliffee N: Effect of alcohol on the individual. *Quarterly J of Studies in Alcoholism* 1940; 1:110–181.
24. Goodwin, DW: Alcoholism and heredity. *Archives of General Psychiatry* 1979; 36:57–61.
25. Hoffman FG: *A Handbook on Drug and Alcohol Abuse,* 2nd ed. New York, Oxford University Press, 1983.
26. Jaffe JH: Drug addiction and abuse. In Gilman AG, Goodman LS, Rall TW, Murad F, eds.: *The Pharmacological Bases of Therapeutics,* 7th ed. New York, Macmillan Publishing Co., 1985, pp. 532–581.
27. Schuckit MA: Alcoholic patients with secondary depression. *Amer J of Psychiatry* 1983; 140(6):711–714.
28. Schuckit MA: The history of psychiatric symptoms in alcoholics. *J of Clinical Psychiatry* 1982; 43(2):53–57.

29. Schuckit MA: Alcoholism and other psychiatric disorders. *Hospital and Committee Psychiatry* 1983; 34(11):1022–1027.
30. Mayfield DG: Alcohol and affect: Experimental studies. In Goodwin DW, Erickson CK, eds.: *Alcoholism and affective disorders.* New York, SP Medical and Scientific Books, 1979, pp. 99–107.
31. Parsons OA, Leber WR: The relationship between cognitive dysfunction and brain damage in alcoholics: Casual or epipheromenal. *Clinic and Experimental Research* 1981; 5(2):326–343.
32. Adams RP, Victor M: *Principles of Neurology,* 3rd ed. New York, McGraw-Hill, 1985.
33. Miller NS, Dackis CA, Gold MS: The relationship of addiction, tolerance and dependence. A neurochemical approach. *J of Substance Abuse Treatment* 1987; 4(3/4):197–207.
34. Lieber CSS: *Medical Disorders of Alcoholism.* New York, W.B. Saunders Co., 1982.
35. Martin RI, Cloninger CR, Guze SB, et al.: Mortality in a follow-up of five hundred psychiatric outpatients. *Archives of General Psychiatry* 1985; 42:47–66.
36. Litman RE, Farberow NL, Wold CI, et al.: Prediction models of suicidal behavior. In Beck AT, Resnick HLP, Lettieri DJ, eds.: *The Prediction of Suicide.* Bowie MD, Charles Press, 1974, p. 141.
37. Dackis CA, Gold MS: Pharmacological approaches to cocaine addiction. *Journal of Substance Abuse Treatment* 1985; 2:139–145.
38. Intergroup Association of Alcoholics Anonymous of Greater New York, 175 5th Avenue, Room 219, New York, NY, 10010.
39. AA General Service Conference. *The AA Member, 1984.* Alcoholics Anonymous World Services. New York, NY, 1984.

11

Outpatient and Inpatient
Treatment of Alcoholism

Surrender to Win

AA SLOGAN

Alcoholism is a chronic disorder associated with progressive medical, psychiatric, and psychosocial dysfunction. Severely addicted patients may require hospitalization before they are capable of recovery. This powerful intervention effectively breaks the cycle of addiction and provides the opportunity to conduct a full medical and psychiatric evaluation under controlled conditions. Coexisting disorders can be identified and treated while the patient is drug abstinent and exposed to rehabilitative treatment. This chapter outlines the inpatient approach to alcoholism and discusses major evaluation and treatment issues.

161

Outpatient Treatment

Purpose

Outpatient drug and alcohol programs were developed to make treatment less costly and more available to individuals in earlier stages of the disease.[7] Like inpatients, participants in intensive outpatient programs are involved in frequent and comprehensive alcohol and drug treatments. Unlike inpatients, outpatients continue their daily involvement at work and at home. Therefore, patients are better able to practice newly learned coping and problem-solving skills on a daily basis with peers and family members. Although inpatient treatment is required for some (especially dependents with concurrent major psychiatric or medical problems), many more people can benefit from the *in vivo* treatment offered on an outpatient basis.

Treatment of drug and alcohol addicts and their family members requires careful planning tailored to the patient. A variety of treatment approaches should be available and applied appropriately to each patient depending on his or her history and needs. The treatment approach offered by most inpatient rehabilitation centers can be made available on an outpatient basis. Some outpatient treatment models are outlined later. But it is important to first consider the assessment process prior to presenting some types and levels of outpatient treatment.

Evaluation and Assessment

A prerequisite for involvement in an outpatient drug and alcohol treatment program is a thorough evaluation and assessment. The evaluation must not only probe drug and alcohol addiction history and prior treatment attempts but also must include a medical history and physical, drug-and-alcohol addiction withdrawal physical examination, psychiatric assessment, and psychosocial evaluation prior to admission. The hospital emergency room is the setting most often used for the evaluation process. But evaluations can also be conducted in a free-standing clinic that has easy access to a hospital for transfer when needed.

Clinic calls are first carefully screened for emergencies. Because patients and family members usually make their first contact for help via telephone, individuals collecting intake information must be knowledgeable about medicine, psychology, and addiction. They must try to find the least invasive treatment setting for the patient's problems *but not* risk the patient's safety. Most patients that call are ambivalent about the need for substance abuse treatment. Therefore, intake personnel must be confident, knowledgeable, firm, and pleasant. In the interest of time, safety, and accuracy, data collection is focused on medical complications of drug and alcohol use (both qualitatively and quantitatively) over the previous few months. Daily opiate, benzodiazepine, or alcohol addicts are often referred for inpatient detoxification, as are intravenous users, crack addicts, polyaddicted, dual-diagnosed, and treatment failures following consultation and confirmation by a medical doctor. Many patients will negotiate toward outpatient detoxification. The hazards, unreliability, and poor outcome of outpatient detoxification should be explained. Patients who do not give a history that clearly warrants inpatient detoxification may be scheduled for an outpatient assessment where the determination can be assessed with more precision. Following detoxification, the patient may require continued inpatient rehabilitation. The detoxed patient may also be referred to a structured outpatient treatment program following detoxification when 24-hour drug and alcohol addiction rehabilitation is not required.

Previous treatment attempts are useful to know about at the time of the initial phone call. Multiple prior outpatient substance abuse treatment attempts may warrant referral to an inpatient drug and alcohol addiction treatment unit or a dual diagnosis treatment center.[4] Never-before treated drug and alcohol addicts should begin on an outpatient basis when appropriate. Even individuals who have been unable to abstain from drugs and alcohol for extended periods of time following multiple inpatient rehabilitation efforts can benefit from an outpatient trial.

Physical Problems and Medications

Physical problems and medications are important to know about at the time of initial contact. Some prescription medications may be dependence-prone drugs that should always be avoided in drug and alcohol addicts. For example, a barbiturate containing medication used for migraine headaches should be replaced by a medication that is not addicting. Use of a beta-blocker or amitriptyline are examples of medical alternatives. Too often, patients are admitted for detoxification and treatment of opiate dependence following extended abuse of pain relievers. These individuals classically have a high tolerance to most other opiate-type prescription pain relievers. Nonaddiction-prone medical alternatives must be made available (i.e., nonsteroidal anti-inflammatory agents) along with physiotherapy or other nonpharmacological methods available to alleviate the pain. In general, severe physical problems associated with drug and alcohol addiction are best managed initially in a hospital setting.

Psychiatric Illness

Major psychiatric illness is an important piece of information to detect during the initial conversation. Alcohol or drug addicts presenting with active major psychiatric illnesses are best treated in an outpatient drug and alcohol addiction clinic only after the psychiatric crisis has been stabilized. Such cases should be referred to more appropriate dual-diagnosis facilities, local inpatient treatment facilities, or an emergency room. The intake person must master the skills practiced by persons working suicide prevention helplines and other crisis intervention and resource hotlines. An appointment for a thorough assessment is made after the initial screening process is complete.

The assessment contains a detailed psychosocial, psychiatric, and drug and alcohol addiction history that typically takes 2 hours. The physician and the assessment counselor then determine the most appropriate treatment for the drug and alcohol addict and his or her family member(s). If inpatient detoxification and rehabilitation is required, then the referral is made and facilitated. If detoxification only is needed, then the patient begins an outpatient program when medically stable. If the patient is in psychiatric crisis, then the crisis is stabilized, and thereafter the need for drug and alcohol addiction treatment is assessed. In most cases, drug and alcohol addicts begin outpatient treatment shortly after the initial assessment if they are not in need of medical detoxification, are not acutely psychotic, suicidal, or homicidal.

Family Programs

Programs for outpatients designed to treat family members of alcohol or drug dependents exist but are scarce. Outpatient drug and alcohol facilities often have family treatment,[5] but too often the services rendered are sparse and infrequent. Although education is important, emphasis is often placed on drug and alcohol addiction issues rather than on the problems experienced by the family members directly. Although a large network of family self-help groups such as Tough Love, Families Anonymous, and Al-Anon[6] exist throughout the country, family members initially contemplating treatment for themselves prefer professional guided individual or group therapy. Family treatment is discussed in a separate chapter of this volume.

Inpatient Treatment

Indications for Hospitalization

Hospitalization for alcoholism is indicated when outpatient treatment has consistently failed or is likely to fail.[1] Severe alcoholism represents a life-threatening situation. Psychiatric disturbances may lead to suicide and dangerously impaired judgment. Accidental death can occur during intoxication states,[2] and medical complications of alcoholism can prove fatal. Given the hazards of alcoholism, hospitalization is a reasonable intervention in cases where absolute control of the patient and his or her environment is necessary.

Alcoholics with serious medical complications are candidates for inpatient treatment. These conditions include overdose, abstinence syndromes, and most diseases related to addiction. Psychiatric illness associated with suicidal, homicidal, or grossly disorganized states obviously requires hospitalization. Under controlled and alcohol-free conditions, certain patients with anxiety and depression may be unable to tolerate outpatient rehabilitation until their psychiatric symptoms are properly evaluated and treated. Inpatient treatment may also be necessary for alcoholics unwilling to leave work or living environments with extraordinary daily access to drugs. Finally, patients averse to treatment but externally motivated by legal, family, or job pressure may develop internal motivation during intensive inpatient rehabilitation.

Evaluation

The optimal assessment of alcoholic patients is conducted on a separate evaluation unit.[3] The evaluation unit addresses intoxication, withdrawal, and coexisting psychiatric and medical disorders that would otherwise be disruptive to a treatment unit milieu. A complete medical and psychiatric evaluation is necessary before evaluation and treatment can proceed. This complex process involves a thorough, integrated, and structured approach from the moment the patient enters the hospital. The physician must be familiar with the pharmacology of alcohol and be able to recognize intoxication and withdrawal states.[2,4] Other medical and psychiatric complications of alcoholism should likewise be familiar to the physician and multidisciplinary staff.

Admission Procedures

Certain basic admission procedures and precautions are advisable once the patient enters the locked evaluation unit. The unit serves to protect each patient from drug access and impulsive departure during his or her most vulnerable period of treatment. Eye contact is maintained until completion of a luggage inspection and body search for hidden alcohol. It is naive to assume that all patients will be sufficiently motivated to enter the hospital without their drug(s) of choice. Vital signs are then measured and communicated to the admitting physician. A urine sample for drug analysis is obtained under direct urethral supervision.[5,6,3] The patient is then examined by the admitting physician with particular attention focused on intoxication and withdrawal signs and conditions to be described further on. Acute overdose syndromes should be rapidly identified and treated medically.[7] A complete medical and psychiatric interview is then conducted and admission orders are written. At this point the patient is oriented to the unit and its rules, and routine eye contact is discontinued.

Unit rules should be promptly stated and conveyed in writing to all patients. The violation of certain rules represents grounds for possible discharge. These include the use of drugs or alcohol, sexual activity, and physical violence on the unit. Patients are also expected to submit random urine specimens for drug analysis upon request and adhere to various medical precautions. All alcohol and drug unit staff are also expected to submit a urine sample for analysis upon request. All visitors must be screened by an alcoholism counselor and may be asked to submit urine samples or be restricted from visiting. This minimizes access to addicted or alcoholic friends or family members who may be likely to bring drugs into the unit or negatively influence the patient. A status system is useful to define graduated privileges and restrict patients to the locked unit who are psychiatrically or medically unstable or at risk of elopement. Unmotivated patients may be restricted as a means of behavioral intervention.

Withdrawal precautions are necessary for all alcohol and drug patients during the first several days. On this evaluation unit where staff to patient is 3:1, close observation is possible. Patients are often dependent upon several drugs and may minimize or withhold information about drug use. This is particularly important with regard to covert alcohol or sedative/hypnotic dependence because of the perils of these abstinence syndromes. If the initial urine demonstrates the presence of sedative/hypnotics, the index of suspicion for sedative withdrawal should be increased. A well-equipped crash cart and emergency-seasoned nurses and physician staff provide an extra margin of safety. Vital signs are monitored at least four times daily, and a tongue depressor is present at the bedside in case of seizures. Observation for seizure and withdrawal symptoms is most effective when the physician and nursing staff are completely familiar with these conditions.

Medical Evaluation

A full medical history and review of systems must be obtained at the onset of treatment. Family or friend informants are useful because patients often minimize or omit crucial medical information. This particularly occurs with questions about drugs abused, medical complications of alcoholism, and abstinence symptoms. Laboratory tests and the physical examination often provide a more objective and accurate evaluation of medical problems. Past medical records should be obtained and reviewed. Alcohol- and drug-related illnesses outlined in the following paragraphs should be promptly identified and treated.

The physical examination on admission first evaluates the possibility of overdose with alcohol and associated drugs. Most patients enter the hospital intoxicated. Any patient with signs or symptoms of imminent respiratory or cardiac arrest is obviously treated supportively and transferred to an intensive care unit. The admitting physician must be familiar with all signs and symptoms of drug overdose, as well as appropriate emergency therapies.

Laboratory testing includes medical admission studies to identify major medical diseases associated with alcohol or drug use. Additional medical testing should be pursued according to the clinical condition of the patient. The supervised urine sample should be analyzed for specific gravity to insure that the patient has not diluted it to avoid drug detection. Modern enzyme radioimmunoassay or gas chromatography/mass spectrometry (GC/MS) screening for drugs may be ordered on admission.[5,3] Patients who demonstrated altered mood, signs of intoxication, or drastic changes in attitudes can be evaluated for covert drug use with blood sample analyzed by GC/MS.

Dietary and dental problems may be found. Dental pain is a frequent complaint of alcoholics during detoxification. Dental problems have often been present for months or years, masked by drug analgesia. The problem may be so advanced that extraction is necessary to avoid acute ulcerative gingivitis.[8] Vitamin deficiency may be specific to drug use or a reflection of poor dietary patterns. Vitamin replacement during the first 2 weeks of hospitalization is probably a prudent precaution.[9]

References

1. Gold MS, Washton AM, Dackis CA: *Cocaine Abuse: Neurochemistry, Phenomenology and Treatment.* NIDA Monograph, 1985, Rockville, MD.
2. Gold MS, Estroff TW, Pottash ACL: Substance induced organic mental disorders. In *Psychiatry Update* 1985; Hales RE, Frances AJ (eds.): APA Press, Washington, D.C., pp. 227–240.
3. Gold MS, Pottash ACL, Estroff TW, et al.: Laboratory evaluation in treatment planning. In *Somatic Therapies.* Washington, DC, American Psychiatric Association, pp. 31–50, 1984.
4. Estroff TW, Gold MS: Psychiatric misdiagnosis. Chapter 2 in Gold MS, Lydiard RB, Carman JS, eds.: *Advances in Psychopharmacology: Predicting and Improving Treatment Response,* Boca Raton, FL, CRC Press, Inc., 1984, pp. 35–66.
5. Pottash ACL, Gold MS, Extein I: The use of the clinical laboratory. In Sederer LI, ed.: *Inpatient Psychiatry Diagnosis and Treatment.* Baltimore, MD, Williams & Wilkins, 1982.
6. Verebey K, Martin D, Gold MS: Interpretation of drug abuse testing: Strengths and limitations of current methodology. *Psychiatric Medicine* 1985; 3(3):287–297.
7. Olson E, McEnrue J, Greenbaum DM: Recognition, general consideration and techniques in the management of drug intoxication. *Heart and Lung,* 1983; 12(2):110–113.
8. Carter EF: Dental implications of narcotic addiction. *Aust Dent J* 1978; 23:308–310.
9. Gold MS, Verebey K: The psychopharmacology of cocaine. In Gold MS, ed.: *Psychiatric Annals* 1984; 14(10):714–723.

12

Treatment of the Dual-Diagnosed Alcoholic Patient

> Anything that can be done chemically can be done in other ways—that is, if we have sufficient knowledge of the process involved.
>
> WILLIAM BURROUGHS

The occurrence of other psychiatric disorders in addition to alcoholism is not particularly common in comparison to the prevalence of psychiatric symptoms caused by alcoholism. The prevalence of alcohol-induced psychiatric syndromes versus idiopathic syndromes occurs because of the overwhelming pharmacological effects of alcohol and the powerful driving force of addiction. However, alcoholics appear vulnerable to developing idiopathic disorders independent of alcoholism with the same frequency as the general population.[15]

Studies of the prevalence of affective disorders in alcoholics do not demonstrate an increased association between alcoholism and idiopathic affective disorders. Although affective states are commonly caused by alcoholism, these alcohol-induced states are to be distinguished from the unipolar depression and bipolar illnesses that arise as genetically independent from alcoholism. The actual prevalence of alcoholism coincidental with affective disorders is statistically calculated to be 1%. This calculation is based on the assumptions that the prevalence of alcoholism is 10% and affective disorder 10%. Because the two are genetically independent, the two are multiplied to arrive at the prevalence of 1%.[16]

The prevalence of psychotic disorders such as schizophrenia among alcoholics is approximately 1%, as it is in the general population. The prevalence of personality disorders is also no greater among alcoholics before the onset of alcoholism than is the prevalence of personality disorders in the general population. The prevalence of anxiety disorders is the same among alcoholics before the onset of alcoholism and the general population. The prevalence rates for psychiatric disorders not induced by alcoholism are not greater among alcoholics than the prevalence rates for psychiatric disorders in the general population.[17]

The treatment of those psychiatric syndromes induced by alcoholism is considerably different than those psychiatric disorders occurring coincidentally with alcoholism. Different clinical courses are to be expected, and different modalities of treatments are employed for each class of disorders. For the most common disorders, affective and anxiety states, and personality disturbances, and the less frequent psychotic states, a systemic and rational approach will adequately and fully treat combinations of psychiatric disorders in the alcoholic.

The addiction to alcohol and its symptoms take priority in the diagnosis in most instances. Once a preoccupation with the acquisition of alcohol, compulsive use of alcohol, and a relapse to alcohol are established, an addiction to alcohol exists regardless of whether a coincidental disorder is present. The addiction to alcohol is not caused by another psychiatric condition.

Depression and anxiety are usually present and at times in sufficient severity to qualify for DSM-III-R diagnosis of affective or anxiety disorder. In most instances, a period of abstinence from alcohol will result in an alleviation or elimination of the symptoms of depression and anxiety, even of the magnitude of a DSM-III-R diagnosis. The time-course may be days or weeks and less commonly months for the disappearance of a major depression or a panic disorder induced by alcoholism. No pharmacological intervention is indicated and is contraindicated at this point for most alcoholics.[18–20]

The long-range treatment of choice is for the involvement in Alcoholics Anonymous for most alcoholics. Although the principles of therapy in AA are spiritual in nature, the techniques are distinctly behavioral. The approach is for the alcoholic to take actions that will eventually result in a change in mood and attitude. This method of treatment for addiction is similar to the methods employed to treat depression before the advent of antidepressants. The depressed individuals were encouraged and in some instances pushed to take actions that resulted in an improvement in their mood.

Recent studies in the various treatment modalities for the treatment of depression have demonstrated that nonpharmacological therapies such as psychotherapy were as effective in alleviating the symptoms of major depression as antidepressants. Although psychotherapy alone is not sufficient to treat an addiction to alcohol, it may serve as an important adjunct to participation in AA. Furthermore, AA is really a form of psychotherapy, administered in a group setting.

Although persistence of affective and anxiety symptoms beyond weeks may still be ascribed to alcoholism, the need for medications such as antidepressants may be indicated for a period of time. Similar guidelines to the use of antidepressants in depressed nonalcoholics may be used for the depressed alcoholic. The length of treatment with the antidepressants would be for 6 months at the usual therapeutic doses. At the end of 6 months, the antidepressant should be tapered over 2 to 4 weeks.

A withdrawal syndrome with the use of antidepressants is to be expected and is reduced with the gradual tapering of the antidepressant. The dependence syndrome associated with antidepressants is anxiety, depression, insomnia, tremor, malaise, and anorexia. The withdrawal may persist for weeks in some individuals but lessens in severity over time. At times the dependence syndrome to antidepressants may be confused with the symptoms of a depression from other causes. Patient follow-up will usually determine if antidepressant withdrawal is the etiology.[21]

Retrospective diagnosis of psychiatric disorders in alcoholic populations is fraught with difficulties. Errors in diagnosis occur in the retrospective analysis of the patient's history for a variety of reasons. The patient must use recall that is distorted by the denial that is associated with alcoholism. Denial is a feature of alcoholism that extends beyond just the accounts of the drinking history but into other aspects of the patient's mental life. The tendency is to deny that alcohol is a problem and to ascribe the consequences of alcoholism to other causes such as coincidental or causative depression.[8]

Moreover, the cognitive state of the chronic drinker is impaired sufficiently to reduce the recall of the actual sequence of events associated with the drinking and occurring before and during the alcoholism. There is another interesting phenomena called "state-dependent" learning in which the alcoholic only remembers the experience surrounding the drinking when actually in the intoxicated state. Otherwise the recollection of factors associated with alcohol consumption including the consequences is missing in the abstinent state. Studies have documented this state-dependent memory with alcohol consumption.[17]

Also, because of diagnostic confusion, many alcoholics who seek treatment for their depression will receive a diagnosis of depression without a proper evaluation of their alcoholism and its role in the depression. Therefore, the alcoholic will have a "dual diagnosis" by history but in fact may only have alcoholism and its attendant consequences. Even obtaining the "old records" will often not be revealing because the alcoholism is not adequately addressed in the previous evaluations.

The existence of a "true depressive or anxiety disorder" coincidental with alcoholism should be treated as any disorder and considered as having the same clinical course and prognosis as an independent disorder. There are some differences in the outcome expectations of treatment in that active participation in AA may result in improved functioning and with fewer signs and symptoms of depression. Moreover, the personality disturbances associated with the depressions are often treated with participation in AA. Therefore, the usual methods of treatment of depressive disorders such as antidepressants and psychotherapy are indicated in alcoholics with coincidental depressive disorders.[22]

The treatment of a psychotic disorder that is coincidental with alcoholism is similar to the treatment of that disorder in the absence of alcoholism. The use of antipsychotic medication is necessary to control hallucinations and delusions of a schizophrenic process in order to increase the compliance with the treatment of the alcohol addiction. A schizophrenic is more likely to be able to comply with the treatment of alcoholism if the psychotic symptoms are also under control. In this instance, the schizophrenia may "trigger" the onset of the alcohol addiction but not cause it. Once the alcoholism is reactivated by the ingestion of alcohol, the addiction resumes as the preeminent disorder in the course of the "dual diagnosis."

The natural history of the schizophrenic syndrome associated with alcoholism is similar to that occurring in the absence of alcoholism. The schizophrenic disease does not appear to have different characteristics whether or not alcoholism exists with respect to the signs and symptoms of schizophrenia. However, as stated, the treatment of the schizophrenia may be affected by the disease of alcoholism. In fact, anecdotal clinical experience suggests that active participation in AA will enhance some of the personality characteristics that are troublesome to the schizophrenic.[23]

Of importance is that the schizophrenic will often have special difficulties in a group-based treatment approach. The personality limitations of the schizophrenic because of the negative symptoms of schizophrenia make interaction in a group intimidating, especially in a confrontational group. Also, the structure and discipline required of the group members are sometimes difficult for the schizophrenic to accept. The poverty of emotions and the inability to form a rapport with others preclude the development of group membership and identification by the schizophrenic. The expectations may be lowered for the schizophrenic, however, and group participation may be possible. Also, the deterioration in personality may not be prohibitive for sufficient participation in the group for treatment of the addiction.

The use of medications in the alcoholic must be done with caution. The alcoholic population is a high-risk population for the misuse of any drug whether it has a high or low potential for abuse and addiction. Medications of any kind carry a relative contraindication in the alcoholic population. There is a hierarchy of risk for various medications and drugs. At one end of the spectrum of risk is the highly addicting stimulants, opiates, and sedative/hypnotics (benzodiazepines), and the other end is acetylacetic acid and acetaminophen. However, any drug including medications carries a risk for addiction, tolerance, and dependence. Antidepressants and certain antipsychotic medications are probably in the middle of the spectrum.

The major reasons for the vulnerability of the alcoholic to other medications are the following. First, the alcoholic is more likely to develop an addiction to drugs because of the already existing addiction to alcohol. Eighty percent or more of the alcoholics under the age of 30 are addicted to at least one other drug or medication. Marijuana is the most common, followed by cocaine, benzodiazepines, and others. Between 25% and 50% of the alcoholics are addicted to benzodiazepines. Second, the drug effect of a medication is troublesome to alcoholics, rendering them more vulnerable to misuse of the medication and/or relapse to alcohol. It makes the acceptance of their alcoholism more difficult and reduces the commitment to recovery and what is necessary to establish that commitment.[24]

Third, the basic defect of the alcoholic is a loss of control over alcohol, which is a drug. This loss of control extends to other populations of drugs and medications, leading to the development of abuse, addiction, tolerance, and dependence.

Fourth, the alcoholic has been searching for a drug solution to his problems through his use of alcohol and other drugs. The "faith in a drug or pill" to solve problems is an obsession that the alcoholic continues to pursue endlessly in spite of adverse and costly consequences. The continuation of the faith in the pill (or medication) will distract the alcoholic from making the necessary changes in his or her personality in order to recover from alcoholism.

Last, there are no pharmacological treatments that are specific for addiction. The addictive behaviors do not respond to medications. The associated consequences from alcoholism such as depression and anxiety do not respond to medications. The benzodiazepines may initially ameliorate the anxiety from alcoholism but tolerance, dependence, and addiction to the benzodiazepines develop readily in alcoholics, resulting in similar adverse consequences from benzodiazepines as from alcohol. Benzodiazepines share crosstolerance and dependence with alcohol.[25]

The personality undergoes a profound change beginning with the initiation of abstinence and the application of the 12-step program of Alcoholics Anonymous. The AA program is specific for addiction. The personality undergoes a fundamental change in attitude that begins with an acceptance of the disease concept of alcoholism and establishing a commitment to recovery. The core personality of narcissism, antisocial, immaturity, and dependence that develops as a result of the addiction to alcoholism is gradually replaced by a more outwardly sensitive, respectful, mature, and independent personality. The basic disturbance in the interpersonal relationship is improved with a premium placed on developing productive and harmonious or at least inoffensive relationships.

The use of psychotherapy to assist in this transformation of personality is legitimate, beneficial, and sometimes indispensable. The form of psychotherapy that is useful in the early stages of recovery is cognitive, "in the here and now," directive, confrontational, and supportive. Insight and long-term directed analytic psychotherapy is not only not useful but may be harmful in the early months of sobriety because the alcoholic is not capable of much insight and often has substantial guilt that would be intensified. However, after a period of sobriety, especially in AA, the psychoanalytic method may be very helpful in determining and resolving long-standing conflicts that may be interfering with a contended and constructive sobriety.

References

1. Schuckit MA: Alcoholism and other psychiatric disorders. *Hosp Community Psychiatry* 1983; 34(11):1022–1027.

2. Powell BJ, Penick EC, Othmer E, Bingham SF, Rice A: Prevalence of additional psychiatric syndromes among male alcoholics. *J Clin Psychiatry,* 1982; 43(10):404–407.
3. Martin RL, Cloninger CR, Guze SB, Clayton PJ: Mortality in a follow-up of 500 psychiatric outpatients. I. Total mortality. *Arch Gen Psychiatry* 1985; 42:47–66.
4. Murphy GF: Suicide in alcoholism. In Roy, A, ed.: *Suicide.* Baltimore, Williams and Wilkins, 1986, pp. 89–96.
5. Schuckit MA: The history of psychotic symptoms in alcoholics. *J Clin Psychiatry* 1982; 43(2):53–57.
6. Adams RP, Victor M: *Principles of Neurology,* 3rd ed. New York, McGraw-Hill.
7. Miller NS: A primer of the treatment process for alcoholism and drug addiction. *Psychiatry Letter,* 1987; 5(7):30–37.
8. Milam JR, Ketcham K: *Under the Influence.* Seattle, WA., Madrona Publishers, 1981.
9. Jaffe JH: Drug addiction and drug abuse. In Gilman AG, Goodman LS, Crall TW, Murad F, eds.: *The Pharmacological Basis of Therapeutics.* New York, Macmillan Publishing Co., 1985, pp. 532–540.
10. Miller NS, Gold MS: Suggestions for changes in DSM-III-R criteria for substance use disorders. *Am J Drug Alcohol Abuse* 1989; 15(2):223–230.
11. Crowley RM: Psychoanalytic literature on drug addiction and alcoholism. *Psychoanalytic Review* 1939; 26:39–54.
12. Mayfield DG: Alcohol and affect: Experimental studies. In Goodwin DW, Erickson CK, eds.: *Alcoholism and Affective Disorders.* New York, SP Medical and Scientific Books, 1979, pp. 99–107.
13. Schuckit MA: Alcoholism and affective disorder: Diagnostic confusion. In Goodwin DW, Erickson CK, eds.: *Alcoholism and Affective Disorders,* New York, SP Medical and Scientific Books, 1979, pp. 9–19.
14. Blankfield A: Psychiatric symptoms in alcohol dependence: Diagnostic and treatment implications. *Journal of Substance Abuse Treatment* 1986; 3:275–278.
15. Helzer JE, Przybeck TR: The co-occurrence of alcoholism with other psychiatric disorders in the general population and its impact on treatment. *J Stud Alcohol* 1988; 49(3):219–224.
16. Schuckit MA: Genetic and clinical implications of alcoholism and affective disorder. *Am J Psychiatry* 1986; 143(2):140–147.

17. Goodwin DW, Guze SB: *Psychiatric diagnosis,* New York, Oxford University Press, 1980.
18. Psychoactive substance use disorders. *Diagnostic and Statistical Manual of Mental Disorders,* 3rd ed. rev. Washington, DC, American Psychiatric Association, pp. 165–185.
19. Schuckit MA: Alcoholic patients with secondary depression. *Am J Psychiatry* 1983; 140:6.
20. Schuckit MA: Dual diagnosis: Substance abuse and anxiety. *The Psychiatric Times,* pp. 20–21.
21. Charney DS, Heninger GR, Sternberg DE, Landis H: Abrupt discontinuation of tricyclic antidepressant drugs: Evidence for a noradrenergic hyperactivity. *Brit J Psychiatry* 1982; 141:377–386.
22. Woodruff RA, Guze SB, Clayton PJ, Carr D: Alcoholism and depression. In Goodwin DW, Erickson CK, eds.: *Alcoholism and affective disorders.* New York, SP Medical and Scientific Books, 1979, pp. 39–47.
23. Wolf AW, Schubert DSP, Patterson MB, Grande TP, Brocco KJ, Pendleton L: Association among major psychiatric diagnoses. *J Consult Clin Psychol* 1988; 56(2):292–294.
24. Miller NS, Mirin SM: Multiple drug use in alcoholics: Practical and theoretical implications, *Psychiatric Annals* 1989; 19(5):248–255.
25. Lader M, Petursson H: Long-term effects of benzodiazepines. *Neuropharmacology* 1983; 22:527–533.

13

Benzodiazepine Use and Addiction among Alcoholics

The devil is most devilish when respectable.
ELIZABETH BARRETT BROWNING

The link between alcohol and benzodiazepines is strong. Approximately half of all alcoholics also are addicted to benzodiazepines, and some 50% of those who use benzodiazepines regularly for medical and nonmedical purposes also are alcoholic. (A majority of them also use other drugs as well, most notably marijuana, cigarettes, and cocaine.)[1,34-42] The pharmacological properties and subjective effects of the two classes of drugs are similar, and both are readily available for nonillicit sources, promoting widespread misconceptions of their dangers and addictive potential.

Because alcoholism and benzodiazepine addiction are so often seen together, it is important for the clinician to

181

possess a basic understanding of the dynamics of benzodiazepine use and addiction. This chapter presents an overview of benzodiazepine use in the United States and current
treatment concepts.

A substantial amount of the medical use of benzodiazepines occurs in populations of alcoholics and drug addicts,
who use them nonmedically according to the surveys. Alcoholics and drug addicts constitute 25% of general medical
populations and 50% of general psychiatry populations. The
contemporary alcoholic is a multiple drug addict, and as
many as 80% of the alcoholics under the age of 30 are addicted to at least one other drug.

Benzodiazepines are a frequently used drug by alcoholics as indicated by clinical practice and studies that reveal
up to 50% of alcoholics use benzodiazepines. Opiate addicts
frequently use high-dose benzodiazepines as studies indicate that 30% to 40% are regular users and are addicted.[35-42]

The presumption is that the physician is in most instances prescribing benzodiazepines for a medical reason,
although the use is often for nonmedical reasons. The symptoms for which benzodiazepines are prescribed are common
consequences of drug abuse, addiction, and dependence.
These are symptoms of anxiety, depression, insomnia, seizures that occur commonly as a direct effect of alcohol, marijuana, cocaine, and heroin. Furthermore, the benzodiazepines themselves produce significant anxiety and depression as a consequence of pharmacological dependence to
them. Considerable confusion can result if proper and accurate diagnosis is not made at the time of prescribing the
benzodiazepines.

History of Benzodiazepines

The benzodiazepines were first introduced in 1960.
Chlordiazepoxide (Librium) was the first of the class that

was created in a deliberate attempt to synthesize a tranquilizer without the sedative properties and abuse, addiction, tolerance, and dependence potential of the barbiturates and other sedative/hypnotic drugs. The popularity of the benzodiazepines rose steadily to a peak period in the mid 1970s when diazepam (Valium) was the most commonly prescribed drug of any kind, more than antihypertensive, analgesic, and other psychotropic medications.[1,2]

The popularity of some benzodiazepines has waned while other benzodiazepines have taken their place. Diazepam's high rank has been replaced by alprazolam (Xanax), and flurazepam (Dalmane) has been replaced by triazolam (Halcion). The benzodiazepines remain popular for a number of reasons that include their wide range of indications and few overdose deaths as well as their addiction and dependence-producing ability. Although the benzodiazepines are prescribed for anxiety disorders, insomnia, seizures, and muscle relaxation, their efficacy for prolonged use in these disorders has not been proven, especially if toxicity and adverse consequences are included in the evaluation.[3,4]

The current evaluations of benzodiazepine use and abuse demonstrate clearly that they produce tolerance and dependence in short- and long-term administration. The development of abuse and addiction is also strongly substantiated, although they are not as easily appreciated and identified because of confusion in diagnosis and treatment of abuse and addiction. Significant problems in definitions, diagnosis, interpretations, and conclusions exist in general practice regarding abuse, addiction, tolerance, and dependence and their relationship to use and symptoms produced by benzodiazepnes. The lack of clarity in defining abuse, addiction and tolerance, and dependence in clinical practice leads to institution and perpetuation of the toxicity and untoward effects of the benzodiazepines.

Many excellent studies and reviews exist that establish the following conclusions: (1) Pharmacological dependence occurs often with benzodiazepines; (2) the dependence follows known pharmacological principles in pharmacokinetic and pharmacodynamic models; (3) the dependence occurs rapidly, within a few weeks; (4) the signs and symptoms of tolerance and dependence are indistinguishable from those present in anxiety disorders except, perhaps, in time course, and (5) long-term efficacy in treatment with the benzodiazepines has not been documented.[5-21] The same reports confirm the following conclusions: (1) The benzodiazepines are not as effective in the treatment of anxiety as once surmised, and alternative methods are equally or more effective; (2) the drugs are not as safe as once considered; (3) other methods to treat anxiety are preferred at least as a first approach, particularly, if the origin of the anxiety is alcohol and drugs; (4) the indications for benzodiazepines are narrower than previously defined; (5) abuse and addiction do occur in greater prevalence than previously considered; and (6) the distinction between medical and nonmedical use is not sharp, and significant overlap occurs.[21-31]

Of paramount importance in understanding the benzodiazepines is that all the benzodiazepines have the same mechanism of action and the effects are similar. The differences in the benzodiazepines are in the intensity of the effects and pharmacokinetic properties. In short, a benzodiazepine is a benzodiazepine, and no significant qualitative difference exists despite almost 30 years of development of new derivatives.

Demographic Profile

Fifty billion doses of benzodiazepine drugs are consumed worldwide each day. Over 2 billion tablets of diazepam alone were prescribed in a single year in the United States. During 1985, in the United States, 3.7 million pills were purchased for 81 million prescriptions; the number of pills equaled 15 per person per year, based on 225 million users. The actual number of users was 25 million so that the average "sale" per person was 148 pills per year.[32,33]

The major prescriber of benzodiazepines is more often general practitioners as defined as internists and family practitioners, followed by psychiatrists, then doctors with other specialties. Psychotropic drugs account for almost one-fifth of all prescriptions in nonpsychiatric populations. The major indications for prescribing the benzodiazepines, such as anxiety, insomnia, seizures, and muscle relaxation, make it a particularly attractive medication to have available for treatment of these conditions.[33]

The principal methods that are used to assess the prevalence of benzodiazepine use are the National Prescription Audit, the National Institute of Drug Abuse (NIDA), the National Household Surveys, and the Drug Abuse Warning Network (DAWN). The current findings are that the benzodiazepines are the most frequently prescribed class of the psychotropic medications, more than other types of psychotropic medications. The peak number of prescriptions was 100 million in 1975, and a relatively stable number of 81 million prescriptions were filled in 1985.[1,34]

The 1985 National Household Survey found that the nonmedical use of tranquilizers use is increasing, in spite of the stability in the prescription rates. The percentage of respondents reporting ever having used a tranquilizer increased from 3.6% in 1982 to 7.1% in 1985. Most of the drugs classified as tranquilizers are benzodiazepines. Of those using tranquilizers in the past year (1985), 17% were ages 12–17, 25% were ages 18–25, 31% were 26–34, and 26% were ages 35 and older. The group was composed of 61% males, 89% whites, 7% blacks, and 4% Hispanics.[34]

The users of benzodiazepine for nonmedical use consisted of multiple drug users. The use of other drugs in the past year was alcohol (95%), marijuana (72%), cigarettes (63%), cocaine (49%), and heroin (2%). The rates of non-

medical use of tranquilizers are higher among young adults
aged 18 to 25 than any other group in the general population. In contrast, the highest rate of medical use of benzodiazepine occurs in the over-age-50 group. Among the young
adults, 18–25 years old, the lifetime prevalence was 12.2%
and ages 12–17 years old was 4.8% in 1985.[1,34]

Although the studies report nonmedical use, the nonmedical use of tranquilizers is difficult to distinguish from
their medical use. A sharp distinction between the medical
and nonmedical use of benzodiazepines is not possible to
make based on the current studies available. In either case,
whether medical or nonmedical use is examined, the physician is generally the source of the benzodiazepines.

Diagnosis

The diagnosis of abuse, addiction, tolerance, and dependence to benzodiazepines requires knowledge of the criteria and clinical characteristics for each. Unfortunately,
these terms have lost rigorous distinctions with usage over
time. Also, different medical disciplines have made addi-
tions or subtractions in meaning for the terms. Finally, the
lay public in attempting to analyze and communicate the
problems surrounding abuse and addiction have used the
terms in arbitrary ways. Pervading all the usages of these
terms is a reluctance to use them in correct ways, at times
when the implications attached to them are undesirable.

Abuse is, by classical definition, use "outside" the normally accepted standard for use in a given population. For
example, an infrequent, transient use of benzodiazepines
with some personal or medical consequence is abusive.
Abuse does not ordinarily include addiction, tolerance, and
dependence, which are terms that describe the occurrence
of definite behavioral and pharmacological developments.
The term *abuse* has taken on the meanings of these other pa-

rameters for drug usage and effects. Abuse is misattributed frequently to describe frank addictive behavior with associated withdrawal symptoms of dependence.[44]

Addiction to benzodiazepines on the other hand is a preoccupation with the acquisition of, compulsive use of, and relapse to benzodiazepines. Compulsivity is use in spite of adverse consequences. Addiction to benzodiazepines by definition extends beyond abusive use into pathological dimensions with predictable consequences from the pervasive loss of control. Abuse may be a prelude to addiction as it indicates some exposure to the drug, and perhaps, evidence of loss of control and use that is not normal by societal standards. Addictive use, however, is not bound by standards of use and transcends social norms by its universal characteristics.[43,44]

Tolerance and *dependence* are pharmacological terms that acquired diagnostic meaning incorrectly with a broad mixture of usage. Tolerance is simply the diminishing effect at a particular dose or amount of drug or increasing amounts of the drug that are needed to maintain the same effect. Tolerance bears no direct relationship to abuse and addiction. Tolerance is a normal adaptation by the body or brain to the presence of the drug. Tolerance is a homeostatic mechanism possessed by the host to maintain physiologic functioning within the normal range. Tolerance is, in a physical sense, a resistance to the effect of the drug to alter the host.[43,44]

Dependence is the withdrawal syndrome that occurs in the abstinent state. The onset of the withdrawal syndrome begins when the drug is withdrawn from the individual. The withdrawal syndrome is referred to as the abstinence syndrome, which is the set of predictable and stereotypic signs and symptoms for a particular drug. Pharmacological dependence is a deadaptation of the receptor sites to the absence of the drug after the adaptation occurred to the presence of the drug. The withdrawal from benzodiazepines is a hyperexcitable state that is opposite to the sedative and in-

TABLE 10. Dose Conversions[a] for Sedative/Hypnotic Drugs
Equivalent to Secobarbital 600 mg and Diazepam 60 mg

Drug	Dose (mg)
Benzodiazepines	
Alprazolam	6
Chlordiazepoxide	150
Clonazepam	24
Clorazepate	90
Flurazepam	90
Halazepam	240
Lorazepam	12
Oxazepam	60
Prazepam	60
Temazepam	90
Barbiturates	
Amobarbital	600
Butabarbital	600
Butalbital (in Fiorinal)	600
Pentobarbital	600
Secobarbital	600
Phenobarbital	180
Glycerol	
Meprobamate	2400
Piperidinedione	
Glutethimide	1500
Quinazolines	
Methaqualone	1800

[a]For patients receiving multiple drugs (e.g., Flurazepam 30 mg/d, diazepam 30 mg/d, phenobarbital 150 mg/d), each drug should be converted to its diazepam or secobarbital dose of diazepam 100 mg/d or secobarbital 1000 mg/d.[52]

hibitory effect of the drugs. The enhancement of the GABA receptors by the benzodiazepines promotes a generalized inhibitory effect. A down regulation or decrease in numbers of GABA receptors that occurs in response to the benzodiazepines is an expression of tolerance. An upregulation or increase in the numbers of GABA receptors occurs as the drug is withdrawn as an expression of dependence.[45,46] The manifestations of dependence to benzodiazepines are the result of the hyperexcitable state that may be a reflection of the reduced numbers of the GABA receptors. The hyperexcitable state produces a broad spectrum of signs and symptoms that include anxiety, panic attacks, hyperactivity, agoraphobia, agitation, insomnia, depression, as well as perceptual abnormalities such as feelings of depersonalization and unreality, frank visual hallucinations, and paranoid delusions. These symptoms are similar to the withdrawal syndromes from alcohol and other sedative/hypnotic drugs but differ in onset and time course. Other less commonly reported symptoms of benzodiazepine withdrawal are the neurological symptoms of paraesthesia and numbness, tremor, muscle stiffness and fasiculations, myalgia, ataxia, blurred vision, hypersensitivity to sound and light, taste and smell. Headache and tinnitus are common; formication and pruritus are not infrequent. Gastrointestinal symptoms include nausea, vomiting, constipation, diarrhea, abdominal pain, and dysphagia; an irritable bowel syndrome may occur. Cardiovascular symptoms may be palpitations, flushing, chest pain, and other symptoms of benzodiazepine dependence are hyperventilation, urinary frequency, urgency and incontinence, loss of libido, generalized malaise, increased respiratory symptoms.[6,47,48]

The dependence takes days and weeks to develop to benzodiazepines. Studies suggest that dependence occurs in the majority of users. The onset of dependence is sooner with the short-acting than the long-acting types as is the onset of withdrawal signs and symptoms. The withdrawal from short-acting benzodiazepines has an onset of signs and symptoms within hours, that is, alprazolam produces anxiety of withdrawal within 2 hours of the last dose, and triazolam produces insomnia of withdrawal within 4 hours of the nighttime dose. The onset of seizures, usually, the generalized tonic clonic type, is 2 to 3 days from the last dose, followed by a delirium in 3 to 4 days. The time course for the longer acting benzodiazepines is anxiety within 1 to 2 days of last dose, seizures within 5 to 7 days, and delirium within 7 to 9 days.[49–51]

The frequency of the signs and symptoms of withdrawal is similar to alcohol. Anxiety is almost always present, with other signs and symptoms less constant and persistent. The frequency and severity of the withdrawal is a function of the dose and duration of the use of the benzodiazepines and more obvious with the shorter acting benzodiazepines. The higher the dose and the longer the use, the more likely the full spectrum of the withdrawal syndrome will be evident.

Although tolerance and dependence to benzodiazepines occur often to both long- and short-acting forms, addiction is not necessarily present unless the criteria for addiction are present. Addiction is diagnosed only if a preoccupation with the acquisition, compulsive use, and relapse to the use of benzodiazepines in spite of adverse consequences can be identified. Tolerance and dependence commonly develop to a wide variety of drugs, including those with a low abuse and addiction potential. Antihypertensive and antidepressants have characteristic signs and symptoms of tolerance and dependence without abusive and addictive use. Caution is urged to taper or gradually withdraw patients to avoid consequences of withdrawal.

Suicide and Drugs

Suicide attempts are commonly associated with the benzodiazepines as confirmed by many studies. Yet benzodiazepines are considered safe with very, very low suicide potential. The DAWN data (Drug Abuse Warning Network, sponsored by NIDA) reveal that 51% of the emergency room visits involving diazepam are related to a "suicide attempt or gesture."[1] Drug overdose is the method of choice in 70% to 90% of suicide attempts. Benzodiazepines have replaced barbiturates as the drugs most commonly used in overdoses in suicide attempts, followed by tricyclic antidepressants, phenothiazines, anticonvulsant and narcotic analgesics for the prescribed drugs. Alcohol and drugs, particularly, those that produce addiction, tolerance, and dependence, are the leading risk factors for suicides in some studies. Benzodiazepines, like alcohol, are central nervous system depressants and produce significant depression, anxiety, and suicidal ideation as a pharmacological consequence.[49,50]

Closer observations with clear criteria of addiction, tolerance, and dependence for benzodiazepines reveal that they are not as safe as once considered and may actually contribute to suicidal potential. Indications that a benzodiazepine user may be addicted or that the suicidal thoughts and actions may be due to the benzodiazepines are derived from observing the behavior of the user. If there is preoccupation with acquiring, continued use, and relapse to benzodiazepines, then addiction is present. If the user refuses or is unable to "come off" the benzodiazepines in spite of the adverse consequences, then addiction is the explanation and not the original or underlying disorder for which the benzodiazepines were described, especially if alternative treatments are refused and untried.

Treatment

The treatment of the abuse, addiction, tolerance, and dependence to benzodiazepines is systematic and effective. No one need suffer morbidity and mortality from benzodiazepines. The first step is to identify which of these is present. The correct diagnosis will determine the efficacy of the treatment.

Abuse usually requires an evaluation and treatment of the precipitating events for the deviant use of the drug. A situational crisis, a chronic condition such as anxiety, insomnia, or pain, a hysterical behavior or misinformed user are some of the more common explanations for abusive use. Information regarding the adverse effects of the benzodiazepines, particularly those leading to the abusive use and instruction for an alternative treatment may be sufficient to end the abusive use.

Addiction usually requires a more complex set of steps, although simple in the conceptual approach. Usually, all that needs to be identified is the preoccupation with, compulsive use, and a recurrent pattern of relapse. Denial for accurate use and consequences is a major obstacle that accompanies an addiction. Denial is an inherent feature of an active addiction to anything, including benzodiazepines. Confrontation with the evidence of the consequences of the addiction is effective in dissipating the denial. A one-to-one interview is ordinarily not sufficient to obtain the full history of the extent and complications to identify the criteria of addiction. Corroborative history from family, physician, and employer is often necessary and helpful to make the diagnosis of addiction.

A thorough history and examination are indicated to make other diagnoses of addiction to alcohol and other drugs. Identification of alcohol and other drugs are important aspects to the treatment. Treatment for addiction can be recommended in gradations. The initial referral may be made to physicians and therapists who are skilled in treating addiction and/or to Alcoholics Anonymous or Narcotics Anonymous. If other psychiatric conditions appear to coexist or if the consequences of the addiction appear especially severe, a referral to a psychiatrist, knowledgeable in addictions, is indicated. Other physical and medical conditions may exist that are associated with the benzodiazepine use, such as chronic pain syndromes that may need further evaluation. Nonpharmacological therapies are preferable for chronic states for those who are addicted to drugs and who appear vulnerable to the general "drug effect" in developing other addictions.

Effective outpatient and inpatient programs are available to treat alcohol and drug addiction. Benzodiazepine addiction lends itself to these programs, particularly, if other drugs and alcohol are used by the benzodiazepine addict. The severity of the addiction is the indicator of whether outpatient or inpatient treatment is needed. The inability to remain abstinent and physical conditions that require close medical evaluation and treatment are the major criteria for selection of inpatient treatment. The supervised environment with a protective structure of an inpatient setting may be required for the achievement and maintenance of abstinence.[51]

Outpatient detoxification is possible in the patient who is addicted to benzodiazepines who can tolerate the protracted and gradual taper over an extended period of time. A prolonged detoxification may be unrealistic because it demands an exercise of control over the drug that the addict often does not possess. Also, a more integrated and effective personality and a cohesive social, family, and employment support may favor outpatient treatment because it provides some external control for the addict and implies some adaptive ability and strength in interpersonal relationships.

The detoxification from benzodiazepines can be simplified and easily applied if basic principles are followed. First, benzodiazepines have cross-tolerance and dependence with each other, alcohol, and other sedative/hypnotic drugs. Any benzodiazepine can be substituted for other benzodiazepines and with barbiturates, so that conversion for equivalent doses can be calculated. Second, a long-acting benzodiazepine is more effective in suppressing the withdrawal symptoms and producing a gradual and smooth transition to the abstinent state. Greater patient compliance and less morbidity will result from the use of the longer acting benzodiazepines.[52,53]

Third, select a benzodiazepine with lower euphoric properties such as chlordiazepoxide, avoiding diazepam as much as possible. Fourth, do not leave prn doses as this will give the addict a choice that is beyond his or her control and will reduce drug-seeking behavior. Withdrawal from benzodiazepines is not usually marked by hypertension and tachycardia as with alcohol so that prn doses are not needed. The anxiety of withdrawal should be controlled with the prescribed taper unless objectively it appears that the doses are too low. Caution is urged at this point as drug-seeking behavior needs to be differentiated from anxiety of withdrawal and the anxiety of another disorder. Only the anxiety of withdrawal when severe need be treated with increased doses of benzodiazepines, although this condition is unusual by detoxification with long-acting benzodiazepines. Alternative methods than benzodiazepines for treating the anxiety of another disorder and drug-seeking behavior are indicated. The prescriber must be in control of the dispensing of the benzodiazepines for withdrawal as the addict by definition is out of control and cannot reliably negotiate in the schedule for tapering.

Fifth, the duration of the tapering schedule is determined by the half life of the benzodiazepine that is being withdrawn. For short-acting benzodiazepines such as alprazolam, 7 to 10 days of a gradual taper with a long-acting benzodiazepine or barbiturate is sufficient; 7 days for low dose use and 10 days for high dose use. For the long-acting benzodiazepines, 10 to 14 days of a gradual taper with a long-acting benzodiazepine or barbiturate is sufficient; 10 days for low dose and 14 days for high dose use. The doses should be given in a Q.I.D. interval. Exact numerical deductions are not needed as the long-acting benzodiazepines accumulate to result in a self-leveling effect of the blood level of the benzodiazepines over time.[52,53]

References

1. DuPont RL, ed.: Abuse of benzodiazepines: The problems and the solutions; A report of the Committee of the Institute for Behavior and Health, Inc. *Am J Drug Alcohol Abuse* 1988; 14(1):1–69.
2. Noyes R, Garvey MJ, Cook BL, Perry PF: Benzodiazepine withdrawal: A review of the evidence. *J Clin Psychiatry* 1988; 49(10):382–389.
3. Top 200 Drugs of 1987. *The American Druggist* 1988; 197(2):36–52.
4. Drug evaluations, antianxiety and hypnotic drugs. Chapter 5, ed. 6, *American Medical Association* 1987; 86–103.
5. Smith DE, Wesson DR: Benzodiazepine dependency syndromes. *J Psychoactive Drugs* 1983; 15(1–2):85–95.
6. Ashton H: Adverse effects of prolonged benzodiazepine use. *Adverse Drug Reaction Bulletin* 1986; 118:440–443.
7. Hallstrom L, Lader M: Benzodiazepine withdrawal phenomena. *Int Pharmacopsychiat* 1981; 16:235–244.
8. Busto U, Sellers EM: Pharmacokinetic determinants of drug abuse and dependence: A conceptual perspective. *Clinical Pharmacokinetics* 1986; 11:144–153.
9. Rosenberg HC, Chiu TH: Time course for development of benzodiazepine tolerance and physical dependence. *Neuroscience and Biobehavioral Review* 1985; 9:123–131.
10. Rickels MD, Case G, Schweizer EE, et al.: Low-dose dependence on chronic benzodiazepine users: A preliminary report on 119 patients. *Psychopharmocology Bulletin* 1986; 22(2).
11. Owen RT, Tyrer P: Benzodiazepine dependence: A review of the evidence. *Drugs* 1983; 25:385–398.
12. Ashton H: Benzodiazepine withdrawal: Outcome in 50 patients. *British J ddiction* 1987; 82:665–671.
13. Lader M: Dependence on benzodiazepines. *J Clin Psychiatry* 1983; 44:121–127.
14. Ashton H: Benzodiazepine withdrawal: An unfinished story. *Br Medical Journal* 1984; 288:1135–1140.
15. Busto U, Sellers EM, Claudio NA, et al.: Withdrawal reaction after long-term therapeutic use of benzodiazepines. *New England Journal of Medicine* Oct. 2, 1986, pp. 854–869.
16. Juergens SM, Morse RM: Alprazolam dependence in seven patients. *Am J Psychiatry* 1988; 145(2):625–627.
17. Lader M: The psychopharmacology of addiction—benzodiaze-

pine tolerance and dependence. In Lader M ed.: *The psychopharmacology of addiction.* New York, Oxford University Press, 1988, pp. 1–13.

18. Murphey SM, Tyrer P: The essence of benzodiazepine dependence. In Lader M ed.: *The psychopharmacology of addiction.* New York, Oxford University Press, 1988, pp. 157–166.

19. Tjiauw-Ling T, Bixler EO, Kales A, Cadieux RJ, Goodman AL: Early morning insomnia, daytime anxiety, and organic mental disorder associated with triazolam. *Journal of Family Practice* 1985; 20(6):592–594.

20. Miller F, Whitcup S, Sacks M, Lynch PE: Unrecognized drug dependence and withdrawal in the elderly. *Drug and Alcohol Depend* 1985; 15:177–179.

21. Tyrer PJ, Seivewright N: Identification and management of benzodiazepine dependence. *Postgraduate Medical Journal* 1984; 60(Suppl 2):41–46.

22. Higgitt A, Golombok S, Fonagy P, et al.: Group treatment of benzodiazepine dependence. *British J Addict* 1987; 517–532.

23. Cappell H, Busto U, Kay G: Drug deprivation and reinforcement by diazepam in a dependent population. *Psychopharmacology* 1987; 91:154–160.

24. Greenblatt DJ, Harmatz JS, Zinny MA, Shader RI: Effect of gradual withdrawal on the rebound sleep disorder after discontinuation of triazolam. *New England Journal of Medicine* 1987; 17:722–728.

25. Fyer A, Liebowitz MR, Gorman JM, et al.: Discontinuation of alprazolam treatment in panic patients. *Am J Psychiatry* 1987; 144:303–308.

26. Rickels K, Case G, Downing RW, Winokur A: Long-term diazepam therapy and clinical outcome. *JAMA* 1983; 250(6):767–771.

27. Lader M: Benzodiazepine dependence. *Neuro-Psychopharmacol and Biol Psychiatry* 1984; 8:85–95.

28. Tyrer P, Rutherford D, Huggett T: Benzodiazepine withdrawal symptoms and propranolol. *The Lancet* 1981; 520–522.

29. Pertusson H, Lader MH: Withdrawal from long-term benzodiazepine treatment. *British Medical Journal* 1981; 283:643–645.

30. Pevnick JS, Jasinske DR, Haertzen CA: Abrupt withdrawal from therapeutically administered diazepam. *Archives of General Psychiatry* 1978; 35:995–998.

31. Lader M, Olajide D: A comparison of buspirone and placebo in relieving benzodiazepine withdrawal symptoms. *J Clin Psychopharmacology* 1987; 7(1):11–15.
32. Tyrer PJ: Benzodiazepines on trial. *British Medical Journal* 1984; 288(6424):1101–1102.
33. Griffiths RR, Sannerud CA: Abuse of and dependence on benzodiazepines and other anxiolytic/sedative drugs. In Meltzer HY, ed.: *Psychopharmacology.* New York, Raven Press, 1987, pp. 1535–1541.
34. *National Household Survey on Drug Abuse:* National Institute on Drug Abuse. Washington, DC, U.S. Government Printing Office, 1985.
35. Chan AWK: Effects of combined alcohol and benzodiazepine: A review. *Drug and Alcohol Depend* 1984; 13:315–341.
36. Grantham P: Benzodiazepine abuse. *British Journal of Hospital Medicine* 1987; 37:999–1001.
37. Ciraulo DA, Sands BF, Shader RI: Critical review of liability for benzodiazepine abuse among alcoholics. *Am J Psychiatry* 1988; 145:1501–1506.
38. Schuster CL, Humphries RH: Benzodiazepine dependency in alcoholics. *Connecticut Medicine* 11–13, January 1981.
39. Perera KMH, Tulley M, Jenner FA: The use of benzodiazepines among drug addicts. *British J Addict* 1987; 82:511–515.
40. Laux G, Puryear DA: Benzodiazepines—misuse, abuse and dependency. *American Family Physician* 1984; 30:139–147.
41. Allgulander C, Ljungberg L, Fisher LD: *Acta Psychiatr Scand* 1987; 75:521–531.
42. Sellers EM, Marshman JA, Kaplan HL, et al.: Acute and chronic drug abuse emergencies in metropolitan Toronto. *International J of the Addictions* 1981; 16(2):283–303.
43. Miller NS, Dackis CA, Gold MS: The relationship of addiction, tolerance and dependence: A neurochemical approach. *J Substance Abuse Treatment* 1987; 4:197–207.
44. Jaffe JH: Drug addiction and drug abuse. In Gilman A, Goodman LS, Rall TW, Murad F, eds.: *Pharmacological bases of therapeutics.* Chapter 23, New York, MacMillan Publishing Co., 1985, pp. 532–581.
45. Haefely W: Biological basis of drug-induced tolerance, rebound, and dependence: Contribution of recent research on benzodiazepines. *Pharmacopsychiat* 1986; 19:353–361.

46. Lader M, File S: Editorial. The biological basis of benzodiazepine dependence. *Psychological Medicine* 1987; 17:539–547.

47. Ryan GP, Boisse NR: Benzodiazepine tolerance, physical dependence and withdrawal: Electrophysiological study of spinal reflex function. *Journal of Pharmacology and Experimental Therapeutics* 1984; 231(2):464–471.

48. Rottenberg H: Alcohol modulation of benzodiazepine receptors. *Alcohol* 1985; 2:203–207.

49. Greenblatt DJ, Divoll M, Abernethy DR, Ochs HR, Shader RI: Benzodiazepine kinetics: Implications for therapeutics and pharmacogeriatrics. *Drug Metab Rev* 1983; 14:251–292.

50. Greenblatt DJ, Divoll M, Abernethy DR, Ochs HR, Shader RI: Clinical pharmacokinetics of the newer benzodiazepines. *Clin Pharmacokinet* 1983; 8:233–252.

51. Greenblatt DJ, Shader RI, Divoll M, Harmatz JS: Benzodiazepines: A summary of pharmacokinetic properties. *Br J Clin Pharmacol* (suppl) 1981; 11:11S–16S.

52. Perry PJ, Alexander B: Sedative/hypnotic dependence: Patient stabilization, tolerance, testing and withdrawal. *Drug Intelligence and Clinical Pharmacy* 1986; 20:532–536.

53. Harrison M, Busto U, Naranjo CA: Diazepam tapering in detoxification for high-dose benzodiazepine abuse. *Clin Pharmacol Ther.* October 1984:527–533.

14

Other Drug Use
among Alcoholics

There is something self-defeating in the too-conscious
pursuit of pleasure.

MAX EASTMAN

General Features

The use and addiction to drugs other than alcohol by alcoholics have always been sufficiently prevalent for clinicians
and researchers to note over the years. The importance of
identifying drug use and addiction in alcoholic populations
is crucial to the clinical diagnosis, prognosis, and treatment
as well as to our research formulation of the etiology and
models for abuse and addiction to alcohol and drugs.

The contemporary alcoholic started with alcohol as the
first drug used but progressed to other drug use at an

alarming rate and to a disturbing magnitude. Most alcoholics under the age of 30 years old use at least one other
drug and more often multiple drugs. The use of the other
drugs is frequently addictive and with similar consequences
to an alcohol addiction. However, a majority of drug addicts
who become addicted to a drug first, later develop alcohol
addiction. Alcohol is not usually the drug of choice but is
used addictively as an adjunct with a drug or in substitution
of a drug.

Surveys and Studies

An arbitrary cutoff between young and old alcoholics is
made at 30 years of age but a gradual transition from common to uncommon drug use by alcoholics as age increases,
perhaps, in roughly a linear progression. The most complete
and cited reference for alcohol and drug use is a monitoring
survey conducted annually since 1975 by the National Institute on Drug seniors who are enrolled at the time of the survey. The 20% of the survey who have dropped out or are
chronically absent are not polled in this survey. These surveys may underestimate drug use as many of these students
probably have alcohol and drug problems that led to their
poor success in schools.

The lifetime use by high-school seniors of alcohol is
93%, of marijuana it is 59%, of cocaine it is 16%, of other
stimulants it is 16%, and of tranquilizers it is 14%. The use
in the last month for the same drugs is 70%, 29%, 5%, 14%,
and 2%, respectively. Another national survey also sponsored by NIDA surveys households in the United States for
drug use by young and old. Similar figures are obtained for
the young, and the inverse relationship between age and
other drug use among alcoholics is illustrated in this survey.

The Drug Abuse Warning Network (DAWN) that records visits to emergency rooms in the United States has

found that alcohol used in combination with other drugs was the most frequently cited and accounted for 24% of all drug-related episodes, excluding those episodes related to alcohol alone for which data were not collected.

A national accounting of youths with alcohol and drug problems in the National Youth Polydrug Study revealed that the mean number of drugs regularly used for the alcoholic youths was 4.4. Marijuana and alcohol were the most frequently used drugs on a regular basis, 86% and 80%, of the sample of 2,750 youths, respectively. Amphetamines had the third highest prevalence at 45%, followed by hashish, barbiturates, hallucinogens, and PCP at 42%, 40%, 40%, and 32% respectively. As far back as 1930, 1940, 1950, 1960, and 1970, alcoholics used other drugs in alarming frequency. Freed reviewed 15,447 cases in 46 studies during those years and found 3,046 alcoholics who were also addicted to another drug or a 20% rate of drug addiction among alcoholics. Some of the same drugs prevalent today were used then, that is, barbiturates, opiates, benzodiazepines, and marijuana.

In large-scale studies of inpatient populations of adult and adolescent alcoholics and drug addicts in various treatment facilities, the number of cocaine addicts with the diagnosis of alcohol dependence was in the 70% to 90% range. Similar studies of methadone and heroin addicts show rates of alcohol dependence between 50% and 75%. Approximately 80% to 90% of cannabis addicts are addicted to alcohol. The prevalence of polydrug use and addiction that includes alcohol is the rule for the contemporary drug addict. The monodrug user and addict is a vanishing species in American culture.

Most studies of both alcoholics and drug addicts indicate that alcohol is the first drug used and often addictively. The natural history of alcohol addiction is highly variable and age dependent. Older alcoholics who are over the age of 30 typically began drinking in adolescence and progressed to diagnosable alcohol addiction in their early 20s. A certain proportion began using cannabis, perhaps, 10% to 20%, in their 20s. Another 10% may begin use of stimulants, including cocaine and amphetamines, whereas 20% may use sedative/hypnotics, predominately, benzodiazepines, barbiturates, and meprobamates. Around 50% may continue their alcohol dependence without significant use of any additional drugs to alcohol.

The alcoholic under the age of 30 has progressed by a different time table according to the general increase in drug use in our culture. Over 80% of these alcoholics are addicted to at least one other drug, usually more than one. A triad of alcohol, marijuana, and cocaine addiction is a regular occurrence among the alcoholics being admitted to inpatient and outpatient facilities. Typically, the younger alcoholic begins using alcohol in early teenage years, around 13 to 15 years of age and progresses to addictive use of alcohol by 15 to 16 years of age. A year or two after the onset of alcohol use, other drugs are tried and some used addictively. These include marijuana, then cocaine, followed by hallucinogens (PCP), benzodiazepines, and barbiturates. The pattern of cocaine use has changed dramatically and continues to do so to the present day, most remarkably, by an earlier age of onset of use. The skillful marketing techniques for the cheaper form of cocaine, "crack," have lured younger individuals to addictive use.

Clinical Diagnosis

Investigations into the utility of the DSM-III-R criteria have confirmed what is occurring among alcoholics. The dependence syndrome as defined in DSM-III-R is used to diagnose all types of alcohol and drug dependence by utilizing the same criteria of addiction, tolerance, and dependence. The findings of this important study supported a common dependence syndrome for alcohol and drugs, particularly, alcohol, opiates, and cocaine.

The practice of multiple drug use by today's addict has many practical implications for diagnosis. The identification of only alcohol in a patient is often tenuous and misleading. Because denial is part of the addictive process, an under-reporting and underestimation of use is to be expected in an clinical interview, especially, if only the alcoholic is inter-viewed. Corroborative sources increase the likelihood of ob-taining a more accurate history but still may not reveal the total pattern and amount of alcohol and drug use. These sources may be family, employer, legal agencies, and urine and blood testing for drugs.

Questions regarding the essentials of diagnosis are dif-ficult to have answered in even the most obvious cases. The criteria for addiction that include a preoccupation with, compulsive use of, and relapse to alcohol and drugs are can-didly denied by many alcoholics and drug addicts who are actively using the alcohol and drugs. Questions regarding the development of tolerance and dependence to alcohol and drugs are equally difficult to have adequately answered. Persistent pursuit of the patient in subsequent interviews and a knowledge of the natural history of alcohol and drug use and addiction will often yield satisfying results if the in-tent is to fully understand the clinical dynamics of the alcoholic.

Multiple drug use will determine the clinical presenta-tion of the acute and chronic intoxication syndromes that the alcohol may present with. A mixture of signs and symptoms may confuse the clinical picture to make the diagnosis of any one drug intoxication difficult as well of other psychi-atric syndromes that may be mimicked by alcohol and par-ticularly drugs.

Treatment

The complete knowledge of all drug use in the alcoholic has important implications in treatment in the acute detoxification period as well as the sustaining of recovery in relapse prevention. Different drugs including alcohol may require individualized detoxification schemes that do not always overlap. The physiological withdrawal from alcohol is treated with benzodiazepines, whereas the delusional and hallucinatory symptoms of PCP are treated with a neuroleptic and opiate withdrawal with clonidine or methadone. Furthermore, the protracted withdrawal from hallucinogens, cannabis, and stimulants may require prolonged pharmacological intervention and supportive care.

The treatment modalities are affected by other drug use, particularly, if alcohol exists as an addiction. Individualized education and support are indicated for specific drugs such as cocaine and opiates. The principles of the abstinence-based treatment program that includes Alcoholics Anonymous will work for the alcoholic who has additional drug addictions. The similarities among the multiple drug and alcohol addictions are greater than the differences so that recovery in self-help groups such as AA and NA is possible and is more the rule than the exception presently. Even individual psychotherapy may involve the core of alcohol and drug addiction and its effects on the mind and behavior.

Genetic Implications

The theoretical implications are most interesting to consider, especially because of the genetic and familial studies of the recent decade. Twin, adoption, familial, and high-risk studies have demonstrated a significant genetic predisposition to alcoholism. Identical twins are more concordant for alcoholism than fraternal twins. The biological parent of an adoptee is a more important determinant of alcoholism than the foster parent who reared the adoptee. Alcoholism runs in families. Fifty percent of the alcoholics have a family history positive for alcoholism. A nonalcoholic child of an alcoholic is more likely to have certain neurophysiological and behavioral manifestations in common with other offspring of alcoholics than with matched controls.

The only corresponding studies that have been performed in drug addicts are investigations in the family history for the prevalence of alcohol dependence in cocaine and opiate addicts. The rate of diagnosis of alcohol dependence in the families of 263 cocaine addicts was slightly greater than 50% or approximately 132 cocaine addicts had at least one first-degree relative with alcohol dependence by DSM-III-R criteria. These figures compare favorably with the familial studies of alcoholism. The high rate of alcohol dependence among cocaine addicts and their families suggests a generalized vulnerability to alcohol and cocaine. The genetic predisposition to alcoholism may overlap or share transmission with cocaine and other drug addictions. Alcohol dependence complicates the addiction to many other drugs as noted previously.

Biology of Addiction

Further theoretical implications of the commonality of alcohol and drug addiction are regarding a neurobiological basis for addiction. The loss of control that underlies all the criteria for addictive behavior is manifested by a drive to pursue, use, and resort to alcohol and drugs repetitively and spontaneously. The mechanisms for such a drive may reside in the limbic system where the substrate for addiction may be located. The limbic structures include the amygdala and septal area for mood, the hippocampi for memory association and the drive states for hunger, libido, and thirst. The reward center is also represented among the limbic structures in the hypothalamus.

The striking features of addiction are subserved by the functions in the limbic system. Alcohol and drugs pro-

foundly alter mood, appetite, and drive states. An association between alcohol/drugs and the drive states may be reinforced by the reward center and recorded as memory by the
hippocampi. The drive states entrain the use of alcohol and
drugs in a fashion similar to their autonomous control over
their functions. The pursuit and use of drugs and alcohol
become as easily stimulated and spontaneous as eating,
drinking, and sexual behavior.

Cocaine may activate the limbic system through stimulation of mood, libido, and the reward center through affecting the dopamine transmission. Opiates through the
endorphins and enkephalins act on the reward center. Alcohol may have a widespread effect on the neurotransmitter
systems in the limbic system. All of the drugs of addiction
affect mood, libido, and appetite. These drugs may also
stimulate the mesolimbic system that may be responsible for
the symptoms of schizophrenia such as hallucinations and
delusions. Finally, all the drugs, including alcohol, suppress
frontal lobe function to produce the impairment in judgment
and insight that is characteristic of drug addiction.

15

Suicide in Alcoholism and Drug Addiction

> He drank, not as an epicure, but barbarously, with a
> speed and dispatch altogether American, as if he were
> performing a homicidal function, as if he had to kill
> something inside himself, a worm that would not die
>
> BAUDELAIRE, writing about Edgar Allan Poe

Suicide in alcoholism and drug addiction has always been common. The association between them has been noted for decades, at least as far back as the turn of the century. Many past studies to the most recent have confirmed that alcohol and drug addiction are major risk factors for suicide and precipitants for suicidal behaviors.[1-3]

The relationship between alcohol and drug use with suicides is because of both a causal and a consequential role for alcohol and drugs. Chronic use of alcohol and drugs has a primary etiologic impact on the emergence of suicidal thinking and actions. The toxic effects of alcohol and drugs on the brain induce suicidal thinking and behaviors by the pharmacological effects that impair judgment and cognition and depress mood. The crisis-oriented life of the addict with disruption of interpersonal relationships is conducive to the development of suicidal impulses, by augmenting the feelings of hopelessness instituted by the addictive process. Moreover, the alcoholic and drug addict may have comorbid psychiatic disorders that also have suicide as a significant risk factor.[4-6]

Prevalence of Suicide in Alcohol and Drug Populations

Alcohol and drug use are associated with 50% or greater of the suicides in either alcoholic and drug addiction populations or nonalcoholic and non-drug-addiction populations.[7-12] Moreover, studies have provided substantial agreement that suicidal behavior including suicides are highly prevalent among alcoholics and drug addicts. These findings of prevalent suicides are derived both from adult and adolescent populations of alcoholic and drug addicts.[13,14] Among adolescents, suicide ranks as the number two cause of death next to accidents. As alcoholism and drug addiction are youthful disorders, it is not surprising yet still disturbing that alcohol and drugs are major causes of suicide among adolescents.[15,16]

The most widely cited study involving drug use in suicides found that 58% of the suicides were associated with a diagnosis of drug and alcohol addiction.[7,14,17] Moreover, approximately 25% or greater of alcoholics and drug addicts kill themselves by various means according to several studies.[5,6,18] Recent investigations performed by the Epidemiological Catchment Area (ECA) have confirmed a lifetime prevalence of 18% for suicide among alcoholics and drug addicts.[19] Some investigators have reported that as many as 70% of adolescent suicides are associated with alcohol or drug problems, often of addictive proportions.[9,15]

The use of alcohol and drugs represents the most common means of inflicting self-harm by the individual attempting suicide whether it be by the addict or nonaddict. The use of alcohol to induce an intoxicated state or as a drug of overdose, and drugs in similar instances of intoxication and overdose, are currently the most prevalent methods for suicide attempts and completions.[7,14,16,17]

In terms of relative risk factors, alcohol and drug addiction are the leading risk factor out of all psychiatric disorders according to many studies. Alcoholism and drug addiction are significantly greater contributors to suicide than other idiopathic psychiatric disorders, such as major depression and schizophrenia. In comparisons of weighted relative risks, depression unrelated to alcoholism was only a moderate predictor of suicidal risks (see Table 11).[20] This is not a surprising observation if alcoholism is factored out of depressive disorders. Thus the suicide rate is significantly lowered because alcoholism is a common illness that produces a potentially reversible depression according to many studies. It is likely that many studies reporting high rates of suicide among affective disorder patients do not separate out alcoholism from the affective disorder. This practice is perpetuated by the propensity for alcoholism to produce affective disorder, particularly depression, as an adverse consequence and the denial of abnormal intake by alcoholics and overemphasis on affective disorder in the etiologic rate of alcoholism.

Clinical Characteristics of Suicidal Alcoholics and Drug Addicts

Although suicide attempts and completions may occur at any age in alcoholics and drug addicts, there are two peak

TABLE 11. Factors Associated with Suicide Risk[a]

Variable in rank order	Content of item
1	Age (45 and older)
2	Alcoholism
3	Irritation, rage, violence
4	Prior suicidal behavior
5	Sex (male)
6	Unwilling to accept help
7	Longer duration of current episode of depression
8	Prior inpatient psychiatric treatment
9	Recent loss or separation
10	Depression
11	Loss of physical health
12	Unemployed/retired
13	Single, widowed, divorced

[a]Modified from Litman RE, Faberow NL, Wold CI, Brown TR: Prediction models of suicidal behaviors. In *The Prediction of Suicide*, H Beck, LP Resnik, DJ Lettieri, editors, p. 141. Charles Press, Bowie, MD, 1974.

periods of increased risk among the young and the old. The young in their 20s constituted two-thirds of suicide completions in a San Diego study. However, in the same study the rate of suicide by alcohol and drug addicts is 60% out of all suicides for ages between 30 and 40 years old.[7,14]

The white male is the most likely race and gender to commit suicide, although the rate for black males is increasing. The older male alcoholic is particularly prone to suicide. Being separated, divorced, or widowed provides a greater risk for suicide as does being unemployed or retired. Poor physical health with an acute or chronic condition also enhances the relative risk (see Table 12).[21]

The duration of 9 years for addiction found in past studies is shorter than other earlier studies that have shown a later onset of suicide in the course of alcoholism.[7,14]

Of importance is that suicide risk is most highly correlated with multiple drug use in the multiple addicted.[7,13] Eighty-four percent of the addicts who committed suicide were both alcoholics and drug addicts. In the study previously discussed, the mean number of drugs used among the suicide victims was 3.6 for the alcohol and drug addicts. The drugs were alcohol, opiates, sedatives, amphetamines, cocaine, and marijuana. Interestingly, phencyclidine and hallucinogens were less represented.

Comorbid psychiatric disorders among the alcoholics and drug addicts who committed suicide were more common in comparison to nonalcoholics and nondrug addicts studies.[7,13] The most common comorbid psychiatric syndromes were depression, borderline personality disorder, mania, and schizophrenia. Family history of depression, suicide, and alcoholism were especially prominent in suicide cases.[13]

In a review of a large number of reports regarding suicide attempts and completion before 1974, the factors associated with suicide risks were ranked in a relative order (see Table 2).[11] The older age as a risk factor is present, indicating that although the older alcoholic may be at significant risk, the younger, multiple-addicted alcoholic is also now relatively more at risk for suicide. Alcoholism was then as now a high-risk factor and as discussed drugs are adding to the risk for suicide.[20]

Prior suicidal behavior is a significant predictor of subsequent suicidal behaviors as is recent loss or separation. Although depression is a commonly cited risk factor for suicide, it appears that depression associated with alcohol and drug use harbors a greater risk. This is understandable in light of the dramatic degree of depression induced by the pharmacological effects of alcohol and drugs. The combination of alcohol and drugs, particularly multiple drugs, leads to a profound depression, with hopelessness and helplessness that are conducive to suicidal thinking and behavior.

TABLE 12. Suicide Rate per 1,000 Population among 3,800 Attempted Suicides, by High- and Low-Risk Categories of Risk-Related Factors

Factor	High-risk category	Suicide rate	Low-risk category	Suicide rate
Age	45 years of age and older	24.0	Under 45 years of age	9.4
Sex	Male	19.9	Female	9.2
Race	White	14.3	Nonwhite	8.7
Marital status	Separated, divorced, widowed	12.5	Single, married	8.6
Living arrangements	Alone	48.4	With others	10.1
Employment status[a]	Unemployed, retired	16.8	Employed[b]	14.3
Physical health	Poor (acute or chronic condition in the 6-month period preceding the attempt)	14.0	Good[b]	12.4
Mental condition	Nervous or mental disorder, mood or behavioral symptoms, including alcoholism	19.1	Presumably normal, including brief situational reactions[b]	7.2
Medical care (within 6 months)	Yes	16.4	No[b]	10.8

Method	Hanging, firearms, jumping, drowning	28.4	Cutting or piercing, gas or carbon monoxide, poison, combination of other methods	12.0
Season	Warm months (April–September)	14.2	Cold months (October–March)	10.9
Time of day	6:00 A.M.–5:59 P.M.	15.1	6:00 P.M.–5:59 A.M.	10.5
Where attempt was made	Own or someone else's home	14.3	Other type of premises, out of doors	11.9
Time interval between attempt and discovery	Almost immediately, reported by person making attempt	10.9	Later	7.2
Intent to kill (self-report)	No[b]	14.5	Yes	8.5
Suicide note	Yes	16.7	No[b]	12.3
Previous attempt or threat	Yes	25.2	No[b]	11.0

[a]Does not include housewives and students.
[b]Includes cases for which information on this factor was not given in the police report.
Table by Tuckman J, Youngman WF: A scale for assessing suicide risk of attempted suicides. J Clin Psychol 1968; 24:17.

According to studies, the feeling of hopelessness correlates highly with suicide.

Mechanisms Underlying Suicide

The state of hopelessness is central to the suicidal state whether drug induced or not. Hopelessness is the most common feeling that appears to precipitate self-inflicted destruction. Apparently, the mind set requires "hope" in order not only to sustain sufficient inertia for survival but to avoid self-extinction.

The type of drugs most often associated with suicidal behavior are the depressants, particularly sedative/hypnotics and opiates. The depressant pharmacological actions of these drugs including alcohol induce a depression that is similar to other depressions, characterized by depressed mood, psychomotor retardation, social withdrawal, guilt, and self-reproach.[5,22]

Convenient to understanding mechanisms underlying suicidal behavior, drugs provide a neuropsychopharmacological model for depression. Chronic alcohol use leads to a deficiency in serotonin, whereas chronic cocaine administration produces a marked depletion of many of the neurotransmitters, including serotonin, norepinephrine, and dopamine. In various studies, using different techniques, all of these neurotransmitters have been implicated in the neurobiology of depression. Antidepressants are purported to work by enhancing the levels of these neurotransmitters in the synapse after acute and chronic administration. This is said to be evidence of their role in depression. The "neurotransmitter hypothesis" provides a common pathway for the development of suicidal states for all the drugs.[23–25]

Other less convincing theories attempting to explain suicidal behavior are that (1) a predisposing personality exists for suicide and (2) alcoholics and drug addicts are "self-medicating" an underlying depression for psychosis that is responsible for the suicidal states.[26]

According to most studies regarding the first hypothesis, no predisposing personality appears to adequately explain alcohol and drug addiction. Alcoholics and drug addicts are derived from every conceivable personality type and possess all personality traits that are present in nonalcoholics and drug addicts. Some personality types are overrepresented among addicts, such as antisocial and borderline personality disorder. However, the evidence clearly supports that in many instances the personality disorder is a consequence of the addiction and that the preexisting personality only increases the risk of exposure to alcohol and drugs, thereby, not conferring a specific vulnerability to the development of alcoholism and drug addiction.[18,27] Many personality theorists would defer the diagnosis of personality disorder in the setting of alcoholism and drug addiction until a prolonged period of abstinence had been achieved, allowing the pharmacological effects of the alcohol and drugs to subside.

The self-medication concept also is not supported by studies that carefully examine the effects of alcohol and drugs on mood and affect. Three groups of alcoholics were given alcohol under experimental conditions: (1) depressed alcoholics, (2) depressed nonalcoholics, and (3) nondepressed nonalcoholics. The depressed nonalcoholics experienced the greatest improvement in mood and affect from the alcohol, whereas the depressed alcoholics experienced the least. The alcoholics appear to use alcohol in spite of the depression (often induced by alcohol) and not because of it.[28]

Other reports from cocaine addicts find they experience their greatest euphoria, often with first use of cocaine. With increasing dose and duration of cocaine use, tolerance to the euphoria from cocaine develops, whereas the toxicity worsens. Eventually, the cocaine addict continues to use in spite of the adverse consequences of severe depression, anxiety, and paranoia inherent in the diminishing euphoria.

If self-medication of underlying depression or psychosis were the goal at some point, the use of alcohol and drugs by the alcoholic and drug addict would cease because the drug-induced depression and psychosis exceeds the original symptoms. Actual use of drug and alcohol may arise initially from attempts to "feel better," but once the addiction sets in, the use no longer is dependent on this motivation as addiction has a life of its own.

Clinical Care and Treatment

In most instances, the comorbid depression, with the concomitant state of hopelessness, will diminish and subside over time with abstinence. In the alcoholic and drug addict, because the depression, paranoia, and anxiety are usually induced by alcohol and drugs, abstinence from alcohol and drugs is essential. However, the tendency to relapse for alcoholics and drug addicts is high so that specific treatment of the addiction that is generating the alcohol and drug use must be instituted.

Generally, hopefulness reappears with prolonged abstinence and specific treatment of the addiction. The suicidal thinking and behavior dramatically improve with abstinence but may persist at chronic, low levels because of prolonged pharmacological effects of the drugs and the degenerated state of the personality and life of the addict. All of the factors often respond to treatment of the addiction, and suicide risk is low for most alcoholics and drug addicts in early recovery in spite of suicidal thoughts. Pharmacotherapy with antidepressants and antipsychotics are not indicated in the vast majority of the cases and may actually be harmful in a population that is vulnerable to drug effects, even those from medications. For those unusual instances where suicidal thinking and depression may persist, the selective use of antidepressants may be indicated.

In obtaining a history from a known alcoholic or drug addict, a careful inquiry into the suicidal state is necessary, including all the known risk factors associated with suicide. The addict may deny both drug use and suicidal ideation and behavior so the corroborative history from family and friends is highly desirable and sometimes necessary. Of critical importance, in the setting of a suicide attempt, is to obtain a careful screening for the presence of alcoholism and drug addiction. Unless alcoholism and drug addiction are identified as etiological agents in the suicidal attempt and properly treated, the likelihood for another suicide attempt is high in spite of specific treatments for the comorbid psychiatric symptoms.

References

1. Frances RJ, Franklin J, Flavin DK: Suicide and alcoholism. *Annals NY Acad Sci* 1986:316–326.
2. Mazuk PM, Mann JJ: Suicide and substance abuse. *Psychiatric Annals 1988* 18(11):639–645.
3. Rushing WA: Individual behavior and suicide. In Gibb TP, ed.: *Suicide.* New York, Harper & Row, pp. 96–121.
4. Ward NG, Schuckit M: Factors associated with suicidal behavior in polydrug abusers. *J Clin Psychiatry* 1980; 41:379–385.
5. Murphy GE: Suicide and substance abuse. *Arch Gen Psychiatry* 1988; 45:593–594.
6. Frances A, Fyer M, Clarkin J: Personality and suicide. *Ann NY Acad Sci* 1986; 487:281–293.
7. Fowler RC, Rich CL, Young D: San Diego Suicide Study: II. Substance abuse in young cases. *Arch Gen Psychiatry* 1986; 43:962–965.
8. Dorpat TL, Riley HS: A study in the Seattle area. *Compr Psychiatry* 1960; 1:349–359.
9. Shaffi M, Carrigan S, Whittinghill JR, et al.: Psychological autopsy of completed suicide in children and adolescents. *Am J Psychiatry* 1985; 142:1061–1064.
10. Barraclough B, Bunch J, Nelson B, et al.: A hundred cases of suicide: Clinical aspects. *Br J Psychiatry* 1974; 125:355–373.

11. Kessel N, Grossman G: Suicides in alcoholics. *Br Med J* 1961; 2:1671–1672.
12. James IP: Suicide and mortality amongst heroin addicts in Britain. *Br J Addict* 1967; 62:391–398.
13. Murphy SL, Rounsaville BJ, Eyre S, et al.: Suicide attempts to treated opiate addicts. *Compr Psychiatry* 1983; 24:79–89.
14. Rich CL, Young D, Fowler RC: San Diego Suicide Study: I. Young vs. Old Subjects. *Arch Gen Psychiatry* 1986; 43:577–582.
15. Brent DA, Perper JA, Goldstein CE, et al.: Risk factors for adolescent suicide: A comparison of adolescent suicide victims with suicidal inpatients. *Arch Gen Psychiatry* 1988; 45:581–588.
16. Martin RL, Cloninger CR, Guze S, et al.: Mortality in a follow-up of 500 psychiatric outpatients: II. Cause-specific mortality. *Arch Gen Psychiatry* 1985; 42:58–66.
17. Rich CL, Fowler RC, Fogarty LA, et al.: San Diego Suicide Study: III. Relationships between diagnoses and stressors. *Arch Gen Psychiatry* 1988; 45:589–592.
18. Vaillant GE: A twelve year follow-up of New York narcotic addicts: I. The relation of treatment to outcome. *Am J Psychiatry* 1966; 122:727–737.
19. Helzer JE, Przybeck TR: The co-occurrence of alcoholism with other psychiatric disorders in the general population and its impact on treatment. *J Stud Alcohol* 1988; 49(3):219–221.
20. Litman RE, Faberow NL, Wold CI, Brown TR: Prediction models of suicidal behaviors. In Beck H, Resnik LP, Lettieri DJ, eds.: In *Prediction of Suicide*. Bowie, MD, Charles Press, 1974, p. 141.
21. Tuckman J, Youngman WF: A scale for assessing suicide risk of attempted suicides. *J Clin Psychol* 1968; 24:17.
22. Mayfield DG, Montgomery D: Alcoholism, alcohol intoxication, and suicide attempts. *Arch Gen Psychiatry* 1972; 27:349–353.
23. Brown GL, Goodwin FK: Cerebrospinal fluid correlates of suicide attempts and aggression. *Ann NY Acad Sci* 1986; 487:175–188.
24. Dackis CA, Gold MS: New concepts in cocaine addiction: The dopamine depletion hypothesis. *Neurosci Biobehav Rev* 1985; 9:469–477.
25. Mann JJ, Stanley M, eds.: Psychobiology of suicidal behavior. *Ann NY Acad Sci* 1986; 487.
26. Khantzian EJ: The self-medication hypothesis of addictive disorders: Focus on lesion and cocaine dependence. *Am J Psychiatry* 1985; 142:1259–1264.

27. Valliant GE: The natural history of alcoholism. Cambridge, Harvard University Press, 1983.
28. Mayfield DG: Alcohol and affect: Experimental studies. In Goodwin DW, Erickson CK, eds.: *Alcoholism and Affective Disorders.* New York, SP Medical and Scientific Books, 1979, pp. 99–107.

16

Fetal Effects
of Maternal Alcohol Use

Baby's brain is tired of thinking,
On the Wherefore and the Whence,
Baby's precious eyes are blinking
With incipient somnolence

JAMES JEFFREY ROCHE

It has been generally accepted that alcohol in heavy doses produces birth defects. In July 1981, the Surgeon General of the United States issued an advisory on drinking during pregnancy: "Each patient should be told about the risk of alcohol consumption during pregnancy, and advised not to drink alcoholic beverages and to be aware of the alcoholic contents of foods and drugs."[1,2,21,22,28]

It is well known that alcohol crosses the placenta barrier freely to reach the fetus. Although it is known that substantial amounts of alcohol intake by the mother can adversely affect the fetus, it is less well known that small-to-moderate amounts of alcohol can lead to dangerous consequences.[5,6,23,24]

Birth weights are lower in infants from mother's consumption of alcohol as small as 30 ml (1 oz) per day, and an increased risk of spontaneous abortions with ingestion of alcohol as little as 30 ml per week, as well as major deformities and impairments that are characterized as the fetal alcohol syndrome (FAS) that is associated with heavy maternal drinking.[3,4,25,26]

Many studies on the fetal effects of alcohol consumption show a positive correlation between maternal alcohol consumption and the risk of fetal abnormalities in any population. These fetal abnormalities may range from selected fetal alcohol effects (FAE) to the full-blown fetal alcohol syndrome (FAS).

The FAS are classified as follows: (1) facial dysmorphology (2) prenatal and antenatal growth deficiency (3) central nervous system involvement, including mental retardation. The FAS occurs throughout the world population in all social strata and ethnicities but is unusually high among American Indians, other lower socioeconomic groups, and children of older mothers.[7,8] Fetal alcohol effects (FAE) are some combinations but not all of (1), (2), (3).

Stillbirths occur more often in women who drink three drinks daily. Spontaneous abortions in the second trimester of pregnancy apparently are three times as frequent in women who have three or more drinks per day as in those who have less than one drink a day. Defective regulation of states of wakefulness and sleep in the newborn also has been attributed to maternal alcohol abuse.[9,10]

Moderate Use of Alcohol

Many methodological problems exist in attempting to determine the effect of moderate alcohol consumption on the fetus. Many of these problems center around the denial and minimization of alcohol use in maternal populations. This is a common problem throughout studies that acquire information on alcohol consumption. Furthermore, the definitions of moderate use vary considerably from 1 to 45 drinks per month. In spite of these problems, investigators have surmised a continuum of increased risks for fetal effects from alcohol in a dose-dependent manner. Fetal abnormalities increased in severity with greater and more frequent doses of alcohol to the full fetal alcohol syndrome. The consequences of alcohol on the fetus may be viewed as a spectrum from minor alterations in development at lower doses and more major abnormalities with major doses and regular consumption of alcohol. For instance, in low-to-moderate doses, fetal alcohol effects (FAE), may be manifested by small size and mental retardation. In heavy doses over prolonged periods during the pregnancy, the fetal alcohol syndrome (FAS) may appear. And any combination of FAE may occur with varying doses and duration of maternal alcohol use during pregnancy. Although the first trimester is the peak period for alcohol toxicity on the fetus to occur, studies indicate that fetal abnormalities from alcohol may occur at any stage in the pregnancy.[11-13]

Duration of Defects and Delayed Effects

The persistence of these effects of alcohol on the fetus has been documented in follow-up studies. The low birth weight and small size tend to persist into early childhood. One of the most disconcerting consequences that persists is mental retardation from maternal alcohol consumption. The second most common known cause of mental retardation is, in fact, maternal alcohol consumption. Obviously, gross abnormalities such as are found in the FAS persist indefinitely and are likely to be lifelong.[14,15]

The number of consequences from fetal alcohol effects (FAE) are probably underdiagnosed because of the non-specific nature of the alcohol-induced abnormalities and the delayed onset of some of the more common and devastating consequences, for example, mental retardation. These findings are combined with the denial and minimization of the alcohol use and degree of consumption by mothers, particularly in the first trimester when the pregnancy may not be known and the amount of drinking is not noted. Of course, the acknowledgement by mothers of self-inducing an abnormality in the fetus by drinking alcohol is a very difficult task for them.[16,17] This assumes that physicians ask about alcohol use in the first place, and whether the pregnancy has been diagnosed.

Confounding Variables

Poor nutrition, other drug use, poverty, and concurrent illnesses are frequently associated with defects in fetal development and with alcoholism. The poor dietary intake may have multiple effects on the fetus. The most common known cause of mental retardation throughout the world is starvation and malnutrition. Starvation and malnutrition are commonly associated with alcoholism and regular and heavy alcohol consumption. These represent alternative explanations for some of the fetal alcohol effects.[18]

Other drugs, particularly cocaine and marijuana, are often taken in conjunction with alcohol. These drugs as well as others may have a profound effect on the developing fetus. A fetal cocaine syndrome similar to the fetal alcohol syndrome has been described. The major effects of cocaine on the fetus are low birth weight, small size, irritability, mental retardation, and poor ability to thrive. The long-term effects of cocaine on the fetus are not known yet, as follow-up studies are needed. However, as with alcohol, many of these effects are likely to persist indefinitely and even lifelong.[19,27]

The frequency of concurrent illness is also higher among alcoholics and drug addicts. Studies have indicated that the immune system of alcoholics is depressed from the direct toxic effects of alcohol and the indirect effects of malnutrition. Infections, especially viral insemination of the fetus, may be more common among maternal alcoholics. Viral infections may produce the nonspecific abnormalities that are found in the fetal alcohol effects.

Drinking Patterns and Behavior

The most pronounced effects have been found to occur with the heaviest and most prolonged maternal drinking. The smallest quantity reported to be associated with FAS was six bottles of beer daily (about 75ml or 2.5 oz of alcohol) consumed throughout pregnancy. The shortest duration of drinking related to FAS was the first 8 weeks of pregnancy only. One study showed that women who reduced their drinking early in their pregnancies had infants with less growth retardation than women who continued to drink excessive amounts. A useful conclusion from the studies is that when drinking occurs, it is probably related to the outcome.[20]

Drinking before recognition of pregnancy has been associated with adverse effects on fetal growth and morphogenesis. Drinking before the onset of pregnancy also appears to have an adverse effect on fetal development. Studies have shown greater fetal abnormalities in mothers who drank more before pregnancy than in alcoholic mothers who abstained during pregnancy.

Studies indicate that the stage of fetal development has a significant effect on the type of fetal abnormality that will arise. In the first trimester, dysmorphology is more likely to occur; in the second trimester, fetal loss; and in the third trimester, impaired intrauterine growth.

In animal studies, the effect of intermittent binge administration as well as regular, constant infusion of alcohol produce fetal abnormalities. Apparently regular and daily alcohol consumption is not necessary for abnormal fetal development.[21]

Beverage Types

There is no definite evidence that beverage type has an influence on the development of fetal abnormalities. The active ingredient, alcohol, appears to be the critical factor in the production of the fetal alcohol effects.

Paternal Alcohol Use

No evidence exists from clinical studies that implicate the consumption of alcohol by the male in humans in the production of fetal abnormalities. Based on animal studies, it has been suggested that lower birth weight and other adverse aspects of fetal development may be due to alcohol's possible secondary effects on the male reproductive function such as lowered resistance to mutagenic toxins in the environment.

Summary of Major Findings and Recommendations of the American Medical Association

1. The evidence is clear that a woman who drinks heavily during pregnancy places her unborn child at substantial risk for fetal damage and physical and mental deficiencies in infancy. Physicians should be alert to signs of possible alcohol

abuse and alcoholism in their female patients of childbearing age, not only those who are pregnant, and institute appropriate diagnostic and therapeutic measures as early as possible. Prompt intervention may prevent adverse fetal consequences from occurring in this high-risk group.

2. The fetal risks involved in moderate or minimal alcohol consumption have not been established through research to date nor has a safe level of maternal alcohol consumption. One of the objectives of future research should be to determine whether there is a level of maternal alcohol consumption below which embryotoxic and teratogenic effects attributable to alcohol are virtually nonexistent.

3. Until such a determination is made, physicians should inform their patients as to what the research to date do and do not show and to encourage them to decide about drinking in light of the evidence and their own situations. Physicians should be explicit in reinforcing the concept that, with several aspects of the issue still in doubt, the safest course is abstinence.

4. Long-term longitudinal studies should be undertaken to give a clearer perception of the nature and duration of alcohol-related birth defects. Cooperative projects should be designed with uniform means of assessing the quality and extent of alcohol intake.

5. To enhance public education efforts, schools, hospitals, and community organizations should become involved in programs conducted by governmental agencies and professional associations.

6. Physicians themselves should take an active part in educational campaigns, such as the National Institute of Alcoholism and Alcohol Abuse. In so doing, they should emphasize the often overlooked consequences of maternal drinking that are less dramatic and pronounced than are features of FAS, which are at least indicated, if not sharply delineated, by some of the research that has been conducted in several parts of the world with diverse populations.[1]

References

1. Council on Scientific Affairs: Fetal effects of maternal alcohol use. *JAMA* May 13, 1983; 249(18):2517–2521.
2. Surgeon General's Advisory on Alcohol and Pregnancy. *FDA Drug Bull* 1981; 11:1–2.
3. Little RE, Graham JM, Samson HH: Fetal Alcohol Syndrome— An open letter to physicians. *AM News,* May 5, 1978, p. 4.
4. Ouellette EM, Rosett HL, Rosman NP, et al.: Adverse effects on offspring of maternal alcohol abuse during pregnancy. *N Eng J Med* 1977; 297:5238–530.
5. Streissgruth AP, Landesman-Dwyer S, Martin JC, et al.: Teratogenic effects of alcohol in humans and laboratory animals. *Science* 1980; 209:353–361.
6. Clarren SK, Smith DW: The fetal alcohol syndrome. *N Eng J Med* 1978; 298:1063–1067.
7. Jones KL, Smith DW: Recognition of the fetal alcohol syndrome in early infancy. *Lancet* 1973; 2:999–1001.
8. Streissguth AP: Fetal alcohol syndrome: An epidemiological perspective. *Am J Epidemiol* 1978; 107:467–478.
9. Kamininski M, Franc M, Lebouvier M, et al.: Moderate alcohol use and pregnancy outcome. *Neurobehav Toxicol Teratol* 1981; 3:173–181.
10. Rosett HL, Weiner L: Identifying and treating pregnant patients at risk from alcohol. *Can Med Assoc J* 1981; 125:149–154.
11. Hanson JW, Streissguth AP, Smith DW: The effects of moderate alcohol consumption drug pregnancy on fetal growth and morphogenesis. *J Pediatr* 1978; 92:457–460.
12. Sokol RJ, Miller SI, Reed G: Alcohol abuse during pregnancy, an epidemiological study. *Alcoholism NY* 1980; 4:135–145.
13. Little RE: Moderate alcohol use during pregnancy and decreased infant birth weight. *Am J Public Health* 1977; 67z:1154–1156.
14. Kline J, Shrout P, Stein Z, et al.: Drinking during pregnancy and spontaneous abortion. *Lancet* 1980; 2:176–180.
15. Silva VA, Larangeira RR, Dolnikoff M, et al.: Alcohol consumption during pregnancy and newborn outcome: A study in Brazil. *Neurobehav Toxicol Teratol* 1980; 2:176–180.
16. Rosett HL, Weiner L, Edelin KC: Strategies for prevention of fetal alcohol effects. *Obstetrics Gynecol* 1981; 57:1–7.

17. Sulik KK, Johnson MC, Webb M: Fetal alcohol syndrome: Embryogenesis in a mouse model. *Science* 1981; 214:936–938.
18. Little RE, Ervin CH: Alcohol and reproduction: Research and clinical issues. In Wilsnak SC, Beckman LJ, eds.: *Alcohol Problems in Women.* New York, Gilford Press, 1983.
19. Little RE, Streissguth AP, Guzinski GM: Prevention of fetal alcohol syndrome: A model program. *Alcohol Clin Exp Res* 1980; 4:185–189.
20. Blume SB: Drinking and pregnancy: Preventing fetal alcohol syndrome. *NY State J Med* 1981; 81:95–98.
21. Burd L, Martsolf JT: Fetal alcohol syndrome: Diagnosis and syndromal variability. *Physiol Behav* 1989, Jul. 46(1):39–43.
22. Waldman HB: Fetal alcohol syndrome and the realities of our time. *ASDC J Dent Child* 1989; Nov–Dec 56(6):435–437.
23. Galea P, Goel K: The fetal alcohol syndrome. *Scott Med J* 1989; Aug. 34(4):505.
24. West J: Fetal alcohol effects: Central nervous system and differentiation and development. *NIDA Res Monogr* 1988; 81:380–386.
25. Russell M: Growing up with fetal alcohol syndrome. *NIDA Res Monogr* 1988; 81:368–378.
26. Sokol RJ, Abel BL: Alcohol-related birth defects: Outlining current research opportunities. *Neurotoxicol Terratol* 1988; May–June:10(3):183–186.
27. Chasnoff IJ: Drug use in pregnancy: Parameters of risk. *Pediatr Clin North Am* 1988; Dec: 35(6):1403–1412.
28. Graber HD: Fetal alcohol syndrome preventable. *NJ Nurse* 1986; Jul-Aug.:16(4):10.

17

Alcohol and Drug Abuse and Dependence in Geriatric Populations

One cannot help being old, but one can resist being aged.

LORD SAMUEL

Prevalence and Patterns of Use

The prevalence of alcohol dependence among the elderly has been determined in systematic epidemiologic studies. The progression of the alcohol dependence according to change in age and the pattern of use has been more difficult to assess in geriatric populations. Although alcohol dependence is a youthful disorder with the most common age of onset of alcohol dependence in adolescence and early adulthood, the onset of alcohol dependence may occur at any age, including during the elderly years, which are recognizable as a second peak in prevalence.[1-3]

The prevalence of drug dependence in the geriatric age group is not as clearly documented as alcoholism, although there is considerable evidence that it is a significant problem, particularly, with prescription and over-the-counter medications. The use of illicit drugs by the geriatric population is generally not a common problem, although similar narcotic and other drugs are obtained by the elderly through prescriptions.[4-6]

The rates of lifetime and recent prevalence of alcoholism and drug dependence have been determined by a national cooperative study in five major cities in the United States. The program is known as the Epidemiologic Catchment Area Program (ECA). The ECA was a combination of five interrelated epidemiologic research studies performed by independent research teams in collaboration with the NIMH. The five major cities were Baltimore, Los Angeles, New Haven, Durham, and St. Louis.[7] The uniqueness of this study was that it determined the prevalence of actual diagnoses according to DSM-III-R criteria, whereas all preceding studies had been based on estimates of consumption and of social, occupational, and health consequences of alcohol and drug use.

Prevalence Rate

Prevalence rates are higher among younger than older ages and among men than women. For men, lifetime prevalence in the youngest age group (18–29 years old) is 27%, 30–44 is 28%, 45–64 is 21%, and 65 and over is 14%. Among women, the highest prevalence rate (7%) is found in the youngest age group (18–29), with a decreasing prevalence— 30–44 at 6%, 45–64 at 3%, and 65+ at 1.5%. Current prevalence rates tend to be highest in the youngest ages and decline in the older groups. Correspondingly, the remission rates tend to rise consistently with increasing age. Although alcohol dependence is a disorder of male predominance, there is substantial evidence that the prevalence for women is increasing dramatically, especially among the youngest ages. Other studies of prevalence report a wide variation of prevalence rates at all ages, mostly because of the inherent bias in the methods for ascertaining prevalence rates that are based on estimates and not actual diagnostic criteria.[8–10]

Age of Onset

In accordance with the prevalence rates, the age of onset of alcohol dependence is at an early age in the lifetime of alcoholics. Almost 40% begin between 15 and 19, and the proportion of cases that have begun by age 30 is more than 80%. For the age group 18–29, the age of onset of alcohol dependence was 17.8 years in men and 18.4 in women; for 30–59, age of onset was 24.2 years in men and 27.3 in women; and 60 +, age of onset was 31.0 years in men and 40.6 years in women.[7]

Duration

The mean duration of the course of alcoholism for those who were still living was at least 5 years for 54% and 11 years for three-quarters of the population. It is important to note that these results are taken from the general population and are very different from those seen in treated patients, who frequently come to treatment for the first time only after many years of alcohol-related problems.

Special Populations

The prevalence ratios are higher for special populations among the elderly. The estimates for the prevalence of alcoholism is 25% to 50% in general medical populations and

50% to 75% in general psychiatric populations.[11,12] The elderly comprise a majority of the general medical populations and a significant proportion of the general psychiatric populations. Furthermore, there is no significant age-related decrease in drinking problems associated with alcohol abuse and dependence in the elderly. Unfortunately, the clinical diagnosis of alcohol and drug dependence in the geriatric population made by clinicians is considerably less than the actual prevalence rates as determined in these studies. The underdiagnosing may be as significant in the elderly as in the younger adult and adolescent populations where underdiagnosing remains considerable.[7]

Early and Late Onset in Elderly Populations

There are two major explanations regarding the distribution of the prevalence and the age of onset of alcohol dependence in the geriatric population. One explanation is that alcohol dependence is a progressive disorder that has a peak prevalence in early to midadulthood.[7] The second explanation is that the prevalence of alcohol dependence has a bimodal distribution with an early onset in midadulthood and a later onset in the 60 and older group.[2] It is informative to examine the natural history of alcohol dependence to ascertain the distribution of the onset and prevalence of alcohol dependence in the elderly.[13]

To begin with, the life expectancy of the alcoholic is approximately 10 to 15 years less than that in the normal population. Therefore, as a generalization, the earlier the age of onset of alcohol dependence, the younger the age of death from alcohol dependence. Clinically, this shortened life span is usually attributed to the medical and psychiatric complications from chronic alcoholism. Moreover, substantial research data exist to document earlier mortality from alcoholism. As mentioned, alcohol dependence is a youthful disorder, with the onset of the majority of cases of alcoholism before the age of 30. The remission rate for at least 1 year of abstinence suggests that the duration of the alcoholism is on the average 5 to 10 years for those who do not seek treatment. However, no data are available that has determined how lasting are the remission rates for this chronic, relapsing disorder and how many return to active alcoholism. Clinically, experience strongly suggests that the relapse rate is high.[7]

When these findings are combined with the occurrence of increasing death rate with increasing age, the obvious conclusion is that there is a steady drop in the prevalence of alcoholics with advancing age. However, there probably exists, although it is not as well documented as the earlier onset of alcoholism, a population of alcoholics who do not begin drinking or at least drinking alcoholically until later life, for example, when children have been raised or the career has been established and more leisure time is available. Advancing age, particularly retirement age, may represent another peak period of exposure to alcohol use, similar to the youthful, adolescent period. Studies have demonstrated that in retirement communities, only 21% of the residents are abstainers compared to 45% in the general population of all ages. The cocktail hour appears to be a focal event in the daily life of many retirement communities. Among these retired, elderly individuals, in and out of these communities, a second population of onset of alcohol dependence probably does emerge to account for the proposed bimodal distribution.[2,13]

Drug Dependence

Also in the ECA study, among those of all ages who do not meet lifetime criteria for alcohol dependence, 3.5% have a diagnosis of illicit drug dependence. Among those with alcohol dependence, the diagnosis of drug dependence was much greater, at 18%. The lifetime prevalence rates for illicit drug dependence according to age are 17% for 18–29 years old, 4% for 30–59, and less than 1% for 60+ years old. The prevalence rates for prescription medications are not available in the ECA studies published thus far.

A similar bimodal distribution may exist for drug dependence for the elderly as with alcohol dependence. As with alcohol, there is a sharp increase and clear predominance of drug use and dependence among adolescents, particularly, for illicit drugs.[7] Because of the same factors contributing to the prevalence of alcoholism, that is, mortality from drug use and aging itself, the life expectancy of the drug-dependent subject is reduced. Furthermore, the natural history of drug use is such that there exists a progressive decrease in drug use and dependence for prescription and nonprescription medications with advancing age, particularly in the elderly.[14,15]

It has been well established that the elderly are the largest users of legal drugs in the national population, accounting for approximately 30% of all prescriptions of any medications.[15] The 1985 National Ambulatory Medical Care Survey of office physicians revealed that at least one drug was prescribed in more than 68% of office visits by patients over the age of 65 years of age.[15] The leading prescribed drugs are cardiovascular, sedative/hypnotics, tranquilizers, and analgesics. Of considerable importance is that it is estimated that 25% of all individuals of geriatric age who use psychoactive drugs risk the development of drug abuse and dependence.[14]

Studies have clearly demonstrated that among the 50% to 75% of the elderly admitted to a general psychiatric hospital that was drug-dependent, half was neither recognized nor detoxified, and some experienced medical complications as a result of underdiagnosis.[12] Female benzodiazepine dependents were less likely to be identified than male alcoholics. In a study of 1,101 noninstitutionalized residents, 40% of the sample were using alcohol and psychotropic drugs.[16]

Multiple Drug Use

The propensity of the elderly to use multiple drugs in addition to the high rate of drug use and combined with their enhanced sensitivity to drug toxicity accentuate the problem of psychoactive drug use among them. It has been reported that as much as 20% of the patients admitted to a general hospital has a drug-induced disorder, and 26% of patients referred to a clinic for a dementia workup had, instead, an adverse drug reaction as an explanation for the mental impairment.

A study of nursing home residents revealed that 50% of them received psychotropic drugs, which were led by tranquilizers, particularly benzodiazepines, sedative/hypnotics, and antipsychotic drugs. Moreover, for elderly living independently, analgesics, anxiolytics, and sedative/hypnotic drugs constitute the greatest source for the development of drug dependence with its consequences. In a recent survey, as many as 33% of chronic daily benzodiazepine users were elderly.[17] The use of benzodiazepines by the elderly is disproportionate to their numbers. In other survey, data from the National Disease and Therapeutic Index indicate that patients 65 and older account for 26% of prescriptions of benzodiazepines written as anxiolytics for anxiety and 40% as hypnotics for sleep.[5]

Physician Is the Source

The source of the drugs is the physician in the vast majority of the cases.[14,15] The general practitioner or primary care physician leads the list of physician types, followed by the psychiatrist. The attitude toward drug abuse and dependence and the prescribing practices of the physician are critical determinants in the frequency and prevalence of drug abuse and dependence in the geriatric population.[14,15]

Over-the Counter Medications

Over-the-counter (OTC) medications constitute a major source of complications from drug toxicity and are drugs that have a significant rate of abuse and dependence. Sixty-nine percent over the age of 60 years old use OTC drugs, 40% are daily users, and 80% of the 69% use alcohol. It is well known that OTC use increases with advancing age, especially in females, as approximately two-thirds of all persons over the age of 60 consume at least one nonprescription drug on a daily basis.[6,18]

The types of OTC drugs used by the elderly frequently are analgesics, laxatives, decongestants containing anticholinergics, antihistamines, ephedrine, caffeine, and antiacids, alcohol-containing drugs such as antitussives, vitamins, and others. The indiscriminate use of these drugs is widespread among the elderly because of a variety of reasons. Many of them are psychotropic medications that are sought as drugs of abuse and dependence, and some are for the treatment of chronic disorders such as pain and arthritis and are taken persistently and are less expensive to obtain without a prescription. They are taken mistakenly because of the reduced cognition and judgment in some of the elderly.[6] Finally, of no small significance is the continuous search by the elderly for the elixir to relieve the suffering and to arrest the advancement of aging through drugs.

Identification and Diagnosis

Dependence Syndrome. The essential features of the dependence syndrome as defined by the DSM-III-R criteria include the behaviors of addiction and pharmacologic tolerance and dependence. The behaviors of addiction are the preoccupation with the acquisition of the drug, compulsive use of the drug, and a pattern of relapse to the drug. The preoccupation is manifested by a persisted drive to acquire the drug, always having the alcohol or drug use as a high priority. Compulsive use is continued use in spite of adverse consequences and may or may not be repetitive use. Relapse to the drug is manifested by an inability to reduce or eliminate the use of the drug in spite of recurrent, adverse consequence.[9,19]

Tolerance and Dependence. Tolerance is defined as a loss of an effect at a particular dose or the need to increase a dose to maintain the same effect. *Dependence* is defined as the onset of withdrawal of stereotypic and predictable signs and symptoms on cessation of a drug. Tolerance and dependence are not essential to the diagnosis of addiction, as the criteria for the dependence syndrome in DSM-III-R may be met without them. Furthermore, tolerance and dependence are not specific for addiction and may occur in the absence of addiction. Tolerance and dependence are particularly poor indicators of "dependence" for the elderly because they do not develop dramatically in the elderly. The ability to develop tolerance and dependence actually diminishes with increasing age. This finding has been confirmed in studies of humans and animals. Finally, tolerance and dependence for some drugs develops minimally to moderately clinically, in all ages, such as to alcohol, anxiolytics, sedative/hypnotics, and others to make them marginal clinical markers.[9,19]

It is important to know that denial is a common accompaniment of addiction, so that obtaining the clinical data to make a diagnosis of drug or alcohol dependence is usually a troublesome task if only the patient's history is used. The patient's behavior regarding alcohol, drugs, and corroborative history from others are the key methods for making a proper diagnosis. Often the patient will minimize or rationalize drug use and the consequences of the alcohol and drug use. Direct confrontation is sometimes helpful in obtaining more information, but sometimes it may anger and alienate the patient. This reaction may be instructive in itself as most nonaddicted people will not mind a sincere inquiry into possible harmful effects from alcohol and drugs.[9,19]

Consequences of Addiction. The diagnosis of both alcohol and drug dependence is made by essentially the same criteria according to the DSM-III-R.[19] The DSM-III-R criteria, however, are difficult to apply in the case of the elderly if the emphasis is on the consequences of the drug use.[19] The consequences for drug use in the elderly are often considerably different than for younger individuals. The elderly do not have the same vulnerability for the development of consequences. For instance, the elderly are frequently not employed, live alone or apart from family involvement, and do not experience significant legal problems as a result of their alcohol and drug dependence. The vast majority of their consequences is restricted to psychiatric and medical problems. Furthermore, some of the more common and troublesome psychiatric and medical consequences from alcohol and drug dependence do not fit precise diagnostic categories and pertain to intrapsychic and interpersonal disturbances that can, nonetheless, impair the individual significantly and severely.

These consequences may appear as magnifications of later life phenomena such as isolation, social withdrawal, loneliness, loss of enthusiasm, feelings of abandonment, hopelessness, helplessness, worthlessness, futility, and desperation. Although these signs and symptoms of intrapsychic and interpersonal relationship difficulties are cardinal manifestations of alcoholism and drug dependence, these are also common accompaniments of the aging process. A clinical caveat is to suspect alcohol and drug dependence when these signs and symptoms are present and not pessimistically pass them off as "aging."

Suicide is a particularly common problem associated with alcohol and drug dependence. Next to advancing age, alcoholism and drug dependence are the greatest risk factors for suicide. The elderly are clearly weighted toward suicide as a complication from alcohol and drug use.[8,12,15]

Psychiatric Complications

The psychiatric complications from alcohol and drug dependence are similar to those found in any population, with some shift in emphasis because of the aging process. Anxiety and depression are common consequences of alcohol and drug dependence. The expression of the central nervous system in response to the effects of the alcohol and drugs is predictable and stereotypic. The depressant drugs such as alcohol, anxiolytics, and sedative/hypnotics produce depression during intoxication and anxiety during withdrawal. The sedation is a function of the intrinsic nature of the depressant drug, whereas withdrawal (dependence) is the discharge of the catecholamines by the sympathetic nervous system. The stimulant drugs such as caffeine and ephedrine produce anxiety during intoxication and depression during withdrawal (dependence) for similar reasons, except withdrawal from CNS stimulants represents a depletion of catecholamines.

The depressant and stimulants in chronic use may produce frank psychotic symptomatology such as delusion and hallucinations. These are particularly troublesome in the vulnerable elderly who may already misinterpret and misperceive because of reduced sensory perception. The delusions are frequently paranoid and terrifying, whereas the hallucinations are more often visual than auditory. The anticholinergic, antihistaminic, and ephedrine drugs are prone to inducing delusions and hallucinations, particularly with chronic administration.

It is important to bear in mind that psychotropic drugs are particularly likely to induce a dementia or delirium syndrome. A compromise of the intellect is always a potential problem when alcohol or an anxiolytic, sedative/hypnotic, anticholinergic, antihistamine drug is used on a chronic basis. These impairments in intellect and memory from alcohol and drugs may be indistinguishable from other causes. Studies of alcohol-induced dementia cite age as the heaviest

risk factor in the severity of the dementia. The older alcoholics sustain a more severe decline in intellect. This is confirmed with CT scans that reveal significant cerebral atrophy
among alcoholics, particularly older alcoholics. Identification
of an alcohol or drug-induced dementia or delirium may prevent costly evaluations for metabolic, structural, degenerative, vascular, infectious etiologies.[9]

Medical Complications

The medical complications from alcohol and drugs are
numerous and are referable to the cardiovascular, gastrointestinal, metabolic, cerebrovascular systems. The psychotropic drugs and alcohol produce acute and chronic effects
on these systems to result in substantial morbidity and mortality. Alcohol by itself leads to hypertension, myocardial
infarction, cardiac arrythmias, stroke, peptic ulcer disease,
immunosuppression, accidents, dehydration, and electro-
lyte abnormalities, just to name some of the complications.[9]

What is perhaps not well appreciated is that some drugs
accumulate by being taken up in the fat and muscle stores
and persist for prolonged periods of time after discontinuation of the dose. Because of slow release over time from the
stores back into blood, the protracted effect of the drug on
cognition and memory as well as mood may be experienced
for weeks to months.[20]

Etiology and Pathogenesis

Biology of Inheritance of Alcoholism. The etiology of alcoholism and drug dependence is not known. What is known
is that alcoholism is an inherited disorder that runs strongly
in families. Twin, adoption, familial, and high-risk studies
clearly demonstrate that the biological background of an individual is an important determinant in the development of
alcoholism.[21] Other factors are operative and pertain to the

exposure to alcohol and drugs and the factors that control the exposure.

Familial Alcoholism. The genetic vulnerability to alcohol may also affect the severity of the course of alcoholism. Those with a family history of alcoholism tend to have an earlier onset and a more rapid course of alcoholism. Familial alcoholics also appear to have a greater number and more serious consequences of alcoholism. According to the bimodal theory of early and late onset, the early-onset alcoholics may have a greater family history of alcoholism that is determined by a genetic basis. The later-onset alcoholics in midlife and geriatric age groups may have less genetic loading, expressed as reduced vulnerability.[21]

Exposure

For the geriatric population, exposure to alcohol is determined by a number of conditions. The availability of alcohol and drugs is a rate-limiting step in exposure and is under the control of the individual ultimately but is influenced by many other factors not under his or her control. For instance, retirement communities have cocktail hours, which are by themselves apparently harmless sources of congeniality and congregation, to aid social interaction. For those who have a vulnerability, repeated exposure to the alcohol creates a risk for developing alcoholism.

Another common example for opportunities for greater exposure to alcohol is the middle-aged or retired person's newfound source of freedom from children, rigors of establishing a career, and greater independence in a marriage relationship. The self-control of avoiding regular use of alcohol may be eased with a sense of fewer responsibilities to inhibit greater use of alcohol. Although many may be able to drink moderately for indefinite periods, there is a substantial proportion of individuals who will develop alcoholism, or about 25% of the adult male population. The number of females who are vulnerable is about 7% but is rising rapidly.[7]

Vulnerability

Although the vulnerability to drug dependence other than alcohol is not as well documented, it does, in many instances, parallel that of alcoholism. Alcoholics have an increased vulnerability to developing dependence to other drugs and do so at a significant rate. Although illicit drug use is low in geriatric age groups, the availability for use of dependence-producing drugs, available through prescriptions and over the counter is not. For the elderly, benzodiazepines, sedative/hypnotics, and analgesics (narcotics) are especially prevalent drugs that are prescribed. Benzodiazepines, and many of the sedative/hypnotics share cross-tolerance and dependence with alcohol and are used interchangeably with alcohol by alcoholics.[20]

Anxiety and Depression as Common Consequences

Many of the signs and symptoms produced by alcohol dependence are also produced by the benzodiazepines and sedative/hypnotic drugs. Anxiety, depression, and insomnia are frequent consequences from chronic alcohol intake of moderate to high doses in most consumers, and in low doses in some. There are symptoms for which benzodiazepines and sedative/hypnotics are frequently prescribed. Unfortunately, although the drugs may transiently relieve these symptoms, as did alcohol at one time, as long as the alcohol dependence continues, the need for the drugs will also continue as well as the consequences of the alcohol dependence.[9,20]

Furthermore, as the benzodiazepines and sedative/hypnotics are used chronically, consequences from the dependence to them will develop. These, interestingly, are indistinguishable from the original target symptoms for which drugs were initially prescribed, namely anxiety, depression, and insomnia. Anxiety, depression, and insomnia are frequently induced by the benzodiazepines and sedative/hypnotics because of the development of pharmacological dependence and addiction and are often worse than the original symptoms. This is a likely outcome whether the cause of the anxiety, depression, and insomnia are alcohol dependence or from some other cause or are idiopathic.[9,20]

Differential Diagnosis

The differential diagnosis of disorders that may mimic alcoholism and drug dependence is limited. Once the behaviors of addiction have been identified, the diagnosis of alcohol and drug dependence can be established. Adverse consequences from alcohol and drug use may arise in the absence of addiction but do so without a preoccupation with acquiring and compulsive use in a pattern of recurrent relapse or an inability to abstain or to reduce the amount and frequency to avoid the adverse consequences. In other words, once an addiction to alcohol and/or drugs is established, no other disorder is needed to cause it, as they are primary disorders that probably have a neurochemical basis.[19]

Because the consequences of alcoholism and drug dependence are frequently psychiatric, that is, anxiety, depression, insomnia, and dementia, as well as medical, for example, hypertension, trauma, peptic ulcer disease, other independent psychiatric and medical disorders are frequently confused with them. A major way of distinguishing the consequences of alcohol and drug dependence from other coexisting disorders is to identify and treat the former and allow for a period of abstinence over time. If the psychiatric disturbances are from the alcohol and drug dependence, they will, after an initial worsening from the acute withdrawal, gradually over time, perhaps, protracted, ameliorate and disappear. If the psychiatric disturbances persist without a significant reduction or increase, then they may be determined as independent and in need of proper diagnosis and treatment.

Treatment

Reduced Tolerance to Drugs. Effective treatments for alcohol and drug dependence exist and are available to the elderly. To be avoided is the attitude that the elderly are too old or too slow to benefit from treatment of alcoholism and drug dependence. The nature and type of the treatment may vary from the usual treatment modalities employed for the younger population. The elderly have physical and psychological differences that require special considerations. The physical characteristics involve the disposition of the drugs. Age-related changes result in increased sensitivity to and prolonged effects from drugs. These age changes are from slowed metabolic breakdown of alcohol and drugs by hepatic enzymes and a decreased lean body mass with a relative increase in body fat, reducing the intravascular volume. Serum proteins are also reduced, and in combination with the previously mentioned factors, contribute to an increased concentration of alcohol and drug in the water compartment. Furthermore, the neuroreceptors are more sensitive to alcohol and drugs with advancing age.[8,11]

As a result, the tolerance to alcohol and drugs is reduced in the elderly and the withdrawal syndrome from the dependence is more severe and prolonged. Typically, the complete withdrawal from alcohol and drugs may take weeks to months, relative to days to weeks in younger individuals. Clinically, this is important as detoxification may take considerably longer and require reduced doses of drugs used for detoxification. Correspondingly, the cognitive improvement, reduction in anxiety and depression, chronic pain, and insomnia from alcohol and drugs may resolve more gradually over an extended period of time. Patience is needed as rapid evaluations are frequently not possible in the population of elderly patients. Hospitalization is often indicated because of the associated medical risks of the elderly for outpatient detoxification from alcohol and drugs. However, in the medically stable, outpatient detoxification is possible and may be desirable.

Effective Treatment for the Elderly

Effective inpatient and outpatient treatment programs for alcohol and drug dependence specifically treat the addiction component that is fundamental to the alcohol and drug use. Treatment programs employing group therapy, oriented toward an Alcoholics Anonymous model are particularly effective. The preferred and most successful approach is abstinence from alcohol and the offending drugs, and all drugs with a liability to produce dependence. Most well-done studies have demonstrated clearly that alcoholics cannot drink alcohol in a controlled fashion. To recommend moderation in alcohol (drugs as well) consumption in the elderly alcoholic is contraindicated. Moreover, the use of benzodiazepines and other sedative/hypnotic drugs is also contraindicated and will frequently induce a relapse to alcohol as well as a dependence to the same drugs.

For persistent insomnia, anxiety, depression, and chronic pain, the use of antidepressants and antipsychotics may be indicated. Important to consider in evaluating these complaints is to always bear in mind that the central nervous system changes that must occur for normal mood and sleep, such as a return of REM sleep, may take weeks and months, and other psychotropic medications may delay the return of these vital functions. Also, those who suffer from addiction (dependence) are prone to use the complaints, anxiety, depression, and chronic pain, as justifications and represent drug-seeking behavior originating from the addiction. Medicating these symptoms should be discouraged and avoided.

Elderly people can do well in traditional forms of long-term treatment for alcoholism and drug dependence such as Alcoholics Anonymous and Narcotics Anonymous. It is important for them to select the types of meetings where elderly populations exist. Otherwise, the principles of these "self-help" groups are as applicable for the elderly as for individuals of other ages.

Additional psychotherapy is often useful in supporting and guiding the elderly alcoholic toward a life without alcohol and drugs. The elderly will respond to confrontation and directive forms of psychotherapy for alcoholism and drug dependence as well or better than the younger addict. Even insightful-oriented psychotherapy may be useful in selected cases.

Prognosis and Outcome

Abstinence as an Indicator. The prognosis for untreated alcoholism and drug dependence in the elderly is poor. Alcoholism and drug dependence are chronic, progressive, relapsing disorders that require continuous treatment for permanent remission. Many alcoholics and drug-dependent individuals can and do stop using for periods of time so that the ability to "quit" is not the measure of the overall prognosis. Rather, the ability to maintain abstinence is the best single predictor of prognosis.

Enabling. The so-called "enabler" is the person or system that allows the alcohol and drug dependence to continue. The enabler in a sense "allows" the alcoholic and drug-dependent individuals to continue to use. Without the enabler, many alcoholics and drug dependents would experience spontaneous remission or seek the necessary treatment. The enablers are many and frequently are family members, physicians, and friends, unfortunately. The enabling is often conscious and unconscious and may represent misguided efforts to help. Treatment for the enabler is available through education, group and individual therapy, and involvement in Al-Anon and NarAnon.[22]

References

1. Cahalan D, Cisin JH, Crossley JM: *American Drinking Practices.* New Brunswick, NJ, Rutgers Center of Alcohol Studies, 1969.
2. Atkinson RM, Turner JA, Kofoed LL, Tolson RL: Early versus late onset alcoholism in older persons. *Alcoholism: Clinical and Experimental Research* 1985; 9:513–515.
3. Clark WB, Midanik L: Alcohol use and alcohol problems among U.S. adults. In *Alcohol Consumption and Related Problems: Alcohol and Health Monograph* No. 1. Rockville, MD: National Institute on Alcohol Abuse and Alcoholism, 1982.
4. Baum C, Kennedy DL, Forbes MB: Drug utilization in the geriatric age group. *Geriatric Drug Use—Clinical and Social Perspectives* 1985; 63–69.
5. Schweizer E, Case WG, Rickles K: Benzodiazepine dependence and withdrawal in elderly patients. *Am J Psychiatry* 1989; 146:529–531.
6. Beers M, Avorn JA, Sounerai SB, Everett DE, Sherman DS, Salem S: Psychoactive medication use in intermediate care facility residents. JAMA 1988; 260:3016–3024.
7. Robbins LN, Helzer JE, Przybeck TR, Regier DA: Alcohol disorders in the community: A report from the epidemiologic catchment area. In *Alcoholism: Origins and Outcomes.* New York, Raven Press, 1988.
8. Atkinson JH, Schuckit MA: Geriatric alcohol and drug misuse and abuse. *Advances in Substance Abuse* 1983; 3:195–237.
9. Hartford JT, Samorajski T: Alcoholism in the geriatric population. *J Am Geriatr Soc* 1982; 30:18.
10. Bienenfield D: Substance abuse in the elderly. In Bienenfield, D, ed., *Verwoerdt's Clinical Geropsychiatry* (3rd ed.), Baltimore: Williams & Wilkins, 1990.
11. Schuckit MA: A clinical review of alcohol, alcoholism, and the elderly patient. *J Clin Psychiatry* 1983; 43:396–399.
12. Curtis JR, Geller G, Stokes EG, Levine DM, Moore RD: Charac-

teristics, diagnosis and treatment of alcoholism in elderly patients. *J Am Geriatri Soc* 1989; 37:310–316.

13. Vaillant GE: *The National History of Alcoholism.* Cambridge, Harvard University Press, 1983.

14. Beardsley RS, Gardocki GL, Larson DB, Itidalgo J: Prescribing of psychotropic medication by primary care physicians and psychiatrists. *Arch Gen Psychiatry* 1988; 45:1117–1119.

15. Koch H, Knapp DE: Highlights of drug utilization in office practice, National Ambulatory Medical Survey, 1985. *Advance Data from Vital and Health Statistics,* No. 134. DHHS pub. no. (PHS) 87-1250. Hyattsville, MD: Public Health Service, 1987.

16. Stephens RC, Haney CA, Underwood S: Psychoactive drug use and potential misuse among persons aged 55 years and older. *J Psychoactive Drugs* 13:185–193.

17. Mellinger GD, Bolter MB, Uhlenhuth EH: Prevalence and correlates of the long-term regular use of anxiolytics. JAMA 251:375–379.

18. Whitcup SM, Miller F: Unrecognized drug dependence in psychiatrically hospitalized elderly patients. *J Am Geriatr Soc.* April, 1987; 35:297–301.

19. Miller NS, Gold MS: Suggestions for changes in DSM-III-R criteria for substance abuse disorders. *Am J Drug and Alcohol Abuse* 1989; 2:223–230.

20. Miller NS, Gold MS: Benzodiazepines. *Am Fam Physician* 1989; 40(4):175–183.

21. Goodwin DW: Alcoholism and geriatrics: The sins of the father. *Arch Gen Psychiatry* 1985; 42:171–174.

22. Miller NS, Gold MS, Cocores JA, Pottash AC: Alcohol dependence and its medical consequences. *NY State J Med* 1988; 88:476–481.

18

Prevention

An ounce of prevention is worth a pound of cure.

BENJAMIN FRANKLIN

Prevention is a subject in medicine that is very similar to alcoholism among the attitudes of the physicians. Unfortunately, too many physicians give up too easily in the battle against the onset of an illness. If a fraction of effort and money that is expended in treatment of illness would be devoted to prevention, perhaps much savings in cost, suffering, and lives might result.

A physician feels compelled to "go all out" to save lives almost irrespective of age and illness and cost, that is, expensive intensive care room treatment, in cases of catastrophic illness, in the very young and very old, and persons whose ages are in between. The attitude is against weighing the cost versus benefit except in extremely compelling cases.

However, prevention is not ordinarily aggressively pursued except in large-scale, community-based operations such as for vaccinations and detection campaigns that may identify a patient population for diagnosis and treatment of an illness, less so to prevent one. Perhaps prevention is so little regarded, paradoxically, because of a high cost-effective ratio. Furthermore, physicians are not well trained in prevention in medical school and specialty training.

Alcoholism is an area of medicine that heretofore has received little time and attention in medical school curricula. Alcoholism has not yet gained full acceptance as an illness or a disease. Physicians still debate whether or not alcoholism (and drug addiction) is a disease. The "disease concept of alcoholism" is still stated instead of merely the disease of alcoholism, finding it necessary to think in conceptual terms, instead of actual disease processes.[1]

The physician is not alone in the sparse recognition of alcoholism (and drug addiction) as diseases. Alcoholism is still popularly regarded as an accepted consequence of something else. Excessive or problem drinking is often denied or attributed to other extraneous or underlying causes. Alcoholism, for most, is not a primary and sufficient illness that involves the relentless pursuit of alcohol in spite of adverse consequences. Drinking is generally regarded as a symptom of something else than a disease by itself.

The public generally does not regard drinking as a potentially catastrophic and fatal health hazard. Alcoholism is probably our number one health problem, especially, if drugs are included as they should be in today's contemporary addict. Yet the American public is saturated with practices and attitudes toward acceptance of an almost unlimited alcohol consumption. It is disturbing to note a society that is saturated with announcements about, advertisements for, and almost unlimited access to, alcohol. The country is currently preoccupied with a "drug problem," that is, cocaine, but appears totally blind to the alcohol problem.

It is impossible to watch a sporting event on television

without feeling or at least seeing driving and forceful entice-
ments to drink beer and to drink more beer. The young of
today must know as much about beer as they do about their
favorite star athletes in order to watch them. Athletes themselves are participants in the advertisements. The heroes of
modern America are rallying the young and old to drink
beer.

The youngsters of today, according to surveys, know
more names of beer and other forms of alcohol than they do
presidents and states in the history and geography of the
United States. Children's minds are permeated with clever
and powerful advertisements programmed by the genius of
Madison Avenue. These somewhat innocent citizens are being bombarded with themes and acts that are designed to
get people (and them) to drink.

The older children and adults who read magazines of all
kinds, including the literary ones, are subjected to persistent and often sexy illustrations of compelling reasons to
drink, that is, drinking is indicative of high society, success,
companionship, intimacy, and power. The back page of *The
New Yorker* frequently has an advertisement for a liquor. The
program for the New York Philharmonic frequently contains
ads for liquor as well. Young people who are encouraged to
learn about and experience higher culture are repeatedly
subjected to exhortations to drink to be more advanced.

There are many more examples in all aspects of American society in which exposure to alcohol is strongly encouraged, in fully acceptably and unqualified endorsements by
those who use the proceeds for financial support. Unfortunately, little consideration and restraint because of the
short- and long-reaching implications are given to the wide
exposure and use of alcohol by all ages.

A useful, pragmatic, conceptual approach for consideration of the prevalence rates for alcoholism (drug addiction) is a simple equation: Alcohol and drug addiction

equals vulnerability plus exposure. The most difficult part of the equation and the first step is to recognize that the problem exists and to what magnitude. Without an accurate assessment of the problem, the solutions are vague and understandably inept.[1,2]

The identification of the addiction appears elsewhere in this book and mostly takes an educational approach and gives an honest appraisal of the problem. The behaviors of alcohol addiction (and drug addiction) are the preoccupation with acquisition of alcohol, compulsive use of alcohol (continued use of alcohol in spite of adverse consequences), and a pattern of relapse or return to alcohol and drugs in spite of adverse consequences. The addiction is recognized by both the presence of alcohol and the negative consequences of the persistent use of alcohol. Without acknowledgment of either, the diagnosis is difficult to make and is many times overlooked. Of course, the risk of incorrectly attributing the consequences to something other than the alcohol is frequently a problem.

The vulnerability to the development of alcoholism has been demonstrated to be genetic, at least, in part. As presented in another chapter, twin and adoption studies and familial and high-risk studies have confirmed that a genetic component is implicated in the transmission of alcoholism. The exact nature of this genetic vulnerability has not been identified, although the studies in high-risk individuals strongly suggest that it has a physical basis. Alcoholics and high-risk individuals appear to have enhanced tolerance to alcohol, manifested subjectively and objectively, and attributable to central nervous system functions, namely brain and brain stem.[1,2]

Most of the same studies have not been performed in drug addicts for the inheritance to drug addiction. However, some familial studies have found that alcoholism is prevalent in the families of cocaine and cannabis addicts, suggesting a genetic link between vulnerability to develop addiction to these drugs and alcohol.

Moreover, the vulnerability portion of the equation does not lend itself to easy manipulation. The genetic vulnerability to alcoholism is changed only after generations of mating perhaps, and no ready and quick solution to altering the genes is currently available—or desirable, for that matter. Education and genetic counseling may have an impact on assortative mating of alcoholics, although this has not been attempted on a large scale. It is not clear that it has been advocated by very many or should be.

However, the exposure portion of the equation is subject to manipulation, although, perhaps, not easily because of recognizable resistance. Exposure is inclusive to cover all the various factors that are contributing to the eventual use of the drug or alcohol by those in particular who are susceptible and possess the vulnerability to develop addiction. Exposure is determined by a large number of influences although these may be categorized under attitudes and practices regarding alcohol and drugs.[3,4]

The attitudes toward the use of alcohol are reflected in virtually every aspect of America's way of life because alcohol consumption is a firmly rooted institution. The permissive attitude toward the use of alcohol is evident in everyday life. It is difficult to describe a drinking behavior or event without some attachment of frivolity and humor. Drinking, even to extreme, is a funny happening. Alcohol is served in many public places, at the White House, at most weddings and funerals and many social gatherings. In fact, it is the exception to not have alcohol available as a part of the event. The public pressure to have alcohol as a part of a social event is large as is the pressure to use alcohol by those attending.

The peer pressure on children in and out of schools is frightening. Children must endure tremendous and often insurmountable pressures from their peers to drink and use drugs. Alcohol is the drug first introduced to the child and is frequently the most often used. Childhood and adolescent alcoholism is common, unfortunately, as many as 25% to 50% of the alcoholics in the United States have the onset of their alcoholism in their teenage years. The combination of peer pressure and widespread exposure to alcohol in advertisements and practices results in the majority of young Americans being exposed often and in large doses to alcohol.

Other commonly expressed factors in exposure are "psychosocial factors." The exposure to alcohol does not depend on psychosocial factors that are distinctive except for some notable conditions. Sociopathic males appear to be more likely to be exposed to alcohol, probably for obvious reasons. Sociopaths appear to be high consumers of alcohol and have high rates of alcoholism. As many as 90% of those incarcerated in prisons are alcoholic, and 80% of the homicides involve alcohol use. Over 75% of the cases of domestic violence involve the use of alcohol, in states of intoxication.[3]

The state of deprivation in economic and social conditions does not seem to be a distinguishing "psychosocial factor" in the development of alcoholism. These psychosocial factors may be more important in the origin of illicit drug use and trade, where profit for drug dealing is present and represents an additional motivation for propagation of drug use.

It is also important to recognize that alcohol is a gateway drug for the use and development of addiction to drugs. Most cocaine and cannabis addicts used and became addicted to alcohol before cocaine and cannabis were tried. It seems that the introduction to drugs other than alcohol is somehow dependent on alcohol. In some ways, alcohol is a conduit to other drug use and addiction. The reasons may lie somewhere in the realization that alcohol is a drug and has similar drug effects to the illicit drugs.

The sharp demarcation between alcohol and other drugs is not readily possible on pharmacological and pathophysiological grounds. The distinction between alcohol and other drugs is a legal and social one and subject to considerable error in conferring greater safety for alcohol over some other drugs.

The manipulation of the exposure portion of the equation is possible and could result in dramatic reduction in the onset of alcoholism and drug addiction. The current changes in attitude and practices toward cigarette smoking provides a model to use for alcohol. Public awareness and attitudes changed sufficiently to finally allow the government to acknowledge that nicotine contained in cigarettes is addicting. Heretofore, public opinion and successful lobbying efforts by the tobacco industry prohibited a realistic appraisal of the magnitude of the cigarette problem. Finally, public sentiment was reflected in new city, state, and federal laws regarding the use and sale of cigarettes.

Some of the more dramatic and effective legislation forbids advertisement on television, restricting smoking in public places, and warns the public of the hazards of cigarette smoking. These and other measures have resulted in significant reductions in the exposure to cigarettes. As a consequence, the use of tobacco has dropped considerably in recent times. A gratifying, corresponding reduction in the adverse consequences of cigarette smoking will certainly follow with the lower rate of addiction to them.

The same paradigm can be applied to alcohol consumption. The public awareness and attitudes toward alcohol can result in a change in practices regarding the sale and consumption of alcohol. The type and amount of advertisement for alcohol beverages can be modified to sane proportions, hopefully eliminated altogether, at least, on television. Restricting the places and hours where alcohol can be purchased and used would reduce consumption rates dramatically. These changes will be brought about by legislation prompted by the public. The lawmakers would never venture such decisions regarding alcohol without a directive from the public.[5]

The lowered exposure would likely result in a reduction of consumption and a subsequent lowering of the prevalence rates for alcoholism and drug addiction. This in turn may lead to a reduction in the exposure to illicit drugs, without alcohol as a gateway to them. The adverse consequences from alcoholism would be fewer and less compelling with a reduction in prevalence.

Physicians must lead the way in the reduction of the destruction caused by alcoholism as they did with cigarette smoking. The physician can play a major role in influencing public awareness and attitudes toward alcoholism. The stigma that still hinders further progress in the diagnosis and treatment of alcoholism may be overcome with physician involvement and leadership.

Without physician support, the cost of alcoholism will continue to mount. Neglect of alcoholism is not benign as it is practiced by many. Honest statements about alcoholism need to be made by physicians. Almost the entire treatment industry for alcoholism grew not only without the physician but in spite of the physician. The lack of physician participation has continued to slow even the enormous progress that has been made in the diagnosis and treatment of alcoholism in the past few decades. There is even a risk that the progress may be reversed without physician support.

References

1. Schuckit MA: Biological vulnerability to alcoholism. *J of Consulting and Clinical Psychology* 1987; 55:301–309.
2. Monteiro MG, Schuckit MA: Populations at high risk—Recent Findings. *J of Clinical Psychiatry* September 1988; 49(9) suppl.:3–7.

3. Proceedings of the National Conference on Alcohol and Drug Abuse Prevention. *Sharing Knowledge for Action.* August 3–6, 1986. U.S. Department of Health and Human Services. PHS. ADAMHA.
4. Smart RG: The impact on consumption of selling wine in grocery stores. *Alcohol and Alcoholism* 1986; 21:233–236.
5. Gertstein D: Alcohol policy: Preventive options. In Grinspoon L, ed.: *Psychiatry Update III.* Washington, DC, American Psychiatric Association, 1984, pp. 359–371.

Index

261